BURNOUT

BURNOUT

WHERE THE HEAD GOES, THE BODY FOLLOWS

ADEL ELSAYED M.D.

Publishing support provided by
Ignite Press
55 Shaw Ave. Suite 204
Clovis, CA 93612
www.IgnitePress.us

ISBN: 979-8-9945985-0-4
ISBN: 979-8-9945985-1-1 (E-book)

For bulk purchases and for booking, contact:

Adel Elsayed
adel.elsayed@thebucketmodel.com
thebucketmodel.com

Library of Congress Control Number: 2026902389

Cover design by Angela Victoria Lupus
Edited by Cathy Cruise
Interior design by Jetlaunch

FIRST EDITION

I've asked God to help me write this book in the best way possible, with the aspiration to help people understand themselves better and gain further strength in battling their daily trials and tribulations. Whatever benefit one gains from this work is from God, and whatever mistakes and shortcomings are from me alone. May God forgive me and bless those who have helped me get here!! Amen.

Acknowledgments

After God, there are many individuals whose influence, encouragement, and presence made this book possible. To my immediate and extended family—your unwavering support, belief, and presence have been the foundation upon which this work was built. From the earliest ideas to the final pages, your encouragement, patience, and strength sustained me in ways both seen and unseen. You have been a constant source of inspiration, motivation, and perspective, reminding me of what truly matters and grounding me throughout this journey. Your role in bringing this work to life is immeasurable, and I am deeply grateful for each of you.

My sincere thanks go to my book coach, Cathy Fyock, whose guidance, expertise, and steady support helped me navigate and bring to life a project of this magnitude. I am equally grateful to Dr. Mitch Heroman, a mentor and friend, for helping me understand the impact this work could have on current and future physician leaders and for validating the growing need for this perspective.

I extend my deepest appreciation to Dr. Isis Marrero and Dr. Christopher Kaliebe for their thoughtful editorial contributions, scientific insights, and guidance in refining this manuscript so it could reach and resonate with a wider audience.

To my teachers, professors, mentors, and colleagues in both engineering and medicine: Thank you for shaping how I think, for challenging me, and for elevating my understanding of the systems and human experiences that gave rise to this book.

I am grateful to the entire team at Ignite Press for its editorial expertise, dedication, and craftsmanship in helping transform this manuscript into a work I am truly proud of.

And finally—though never last in my heart—I thank my patients. Your courage, trust, and willingness to allow me into your stories have shaped my purpose since the beginning. You inspired my early desire to engineer better systems for care and later motivated my decision to become a physician, bringing me closer to your journeys. Being part of your healing, in moments of struggle and strength alike, has been a privilege. You planted the earliest seeds of this book, and my hope is that its fruits serve you—and humanity—well.

Table of Contents

Introduction: Time for a Rescue!

Burnout doesn't always announce itself. It doesn't necessarily arrive with a dramatic collapse or a moment of crisis in the middle of your workday. More often, it builds slowly and quietly. It settles in layer by layer, until one day you realize something isn't right—you're not okay. You find yourself moving through the day in a fog. The energy you once brought to your work feels harder to harness. Tasks that once gave you a sense of purpose now feel like obligations. You sleep, but never feel truly rested. Your patience runs thin, and your motivation fades and returns in unpredictable waves. Maybe you've noticed yourself zoning out during conversations or losing track of even simple tasks. You might start questioning your own effort, wondering if the problem is that you're just not trying hard enough.

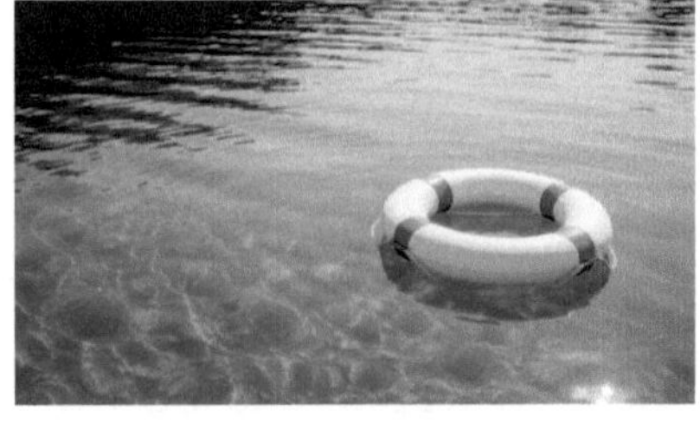

But this isn't about weakness. This isn't about your inability to manage. This is what it feels like when you're underwater. Burnout often creeps in unnoticed until it fills the entire room. On the outside, you may still look composed and capable. But on the inside, everything feels heavy, disconnected, and hard to hold together. The longer you try to dismiss the signs, the harder it becomes to catch your breath again.[1]

There's a principle from lifeguard rescue training that always stuck with me: *Where the head goes, the body follows*. In the water, rescuing someone starts with stabilizing their head—not because the rest doesn't matter, but because if the head is flailing or sinking, the body can't be safely led to shore.[2] But if you can support the head—keep it above the surface and steady the panic—you can guide the rest to safety. Clarity returns. Breathing steadies. That's where the rescue begins. That same principle applies to burnout recovery. It starts with the head—with finding stillness and clarity amid the mental and emotional chaos.

Before I went into medicine, I was trained as an engineer. I've always found comfort in systems—understanding how they function, where they fail, and what it takes to restore them. That mindset shaped how I understand burnout. Burnout isn't just an emotional experience; it's a systemic one.[3,4,5] It's biological, environmental, behavioral, and often cumulative. It doesn't arise from just one thing—it emerges from layers of pressure, compounded over time. It's not always about a toxic job or a single major event. Sometimes, it's the gradual buildup of tension that slowly erodes your capacity to recover.

Burnout isn't just an emotional experience; it's a systemic one.

The scale of the challenge is neither hypothetical nor marginal—it is both real and costly. Globally, depression and anxiety—often downstream of chronic workplace stress and burnout—are responsible for an estimated 12 billion lost working days each year, translating to a $1 trillion cost in lost productivity worldwide.[6] In the United States, workers who report fair or poor mental health miss nearly 12 unplanned workdays annually compared with about 2.5 days for those with good to excellent mental health; overall, poor employee mental health costs the US economy approximately $47.6 billion per year.[7] Within high-demand professions, the burden is still greater. More than half of US physicians report at least one symptom of burnout—nearly twice the rate of the general working population—and physician burnout alone costs the US healthcare system around $4.6 billion annually through turnover and reduced clinical hours.[8] Frontline workers across diverse sectors face similarly alarming trends: Between 2018 and 2022, the proportion of healthcare workers reporting feeling burnt out "often or very often" rose from 32–46 percent.[9] These figures represent not just organizational losses, but human ones—lost engagement; increased error rates; prolonged recovery; erosion of compassion; illness; and, at times, crisis. The ripple effects extend far beyond one individual's experience, undermining teams, institutions, and the very systems we rely on in moments of need.

The idea for this book began with a sketch—a simple drawing of how stress, capacity, and recovery interact like a system. Those first sketches turned into pages of notes, diagrams, and reflections. Over time, they became a binder full of observations drawn from personal experience, clinical practice, and hundreds of conversations with patients, colleagues, and community members. I saw how powerful it could be to offer someone a visual, a metaphor, or a framework that helped them name what they were feeling. I recognized my own story in those conversations too—moments when I had ignored my limits, when I had let the inputs pile up without checking the drains. Writing this book became a way to organize those insights and share them more broadly—with people who need a way to make sense of what they're carrying.

Many models have attempted to define and dissect burnout over the years, each adding something essential to the conversation. The Maslach Burnout Inventory, first developed by psychologist Christina Maslach in the 1980s, gave us the language of emotional exhaustion, depersonalization, and reduced personal accomplishment,[10] though it largely framed burnout in occupational terms. The Job Demands–Resources model reframed burnout as an imbalance between workload and available supports,[11] but it often stayed rooted in organizational structures more than personal experience. Cognitive theories such as Ursin and Eriksen's Cognitive Activation Theory of Stress (CATS) emphasized the role of perceived control and sustained arousal,[12] while newer measures like the Burnout Assessment Tool (BAT)[13] offered diagnostic refinements. Each has value, but many remain either too abstract, too academic, or too far removed from the lived experience of burnout and recovery.

Alongside these, clinicians have long used metaphors like the Stress Bucket Model, which depicts stress as water filling a bucket that eventually overflows unless healthy "taps" or coping outlets are opened.[14] This simple visual has been invaluable in education and therapy because it makes an invisible process feel concrete. Yet its focus is mostly on stress and coping in broad terms, without fully accounting for the interplay of biology, trauma, social determinants of health, or the subtle accumulation that leads to burnout.[15]

In this book, we build on these various theories and concepts, while providing a more tangible, applicable, and comprehensive view of burnout, the various reasons that lead to it, and how to potentially manage it. It doesn't replace existing theories—it extends them. It offers not only explanation but direction, helping people locate themselves in the burnout equation and identify levers they can actually adjust.

This book is for people who shoulder a lot. Leaders, parents, caretakers, educators, healthcare professionals, first responders—anyone who performs under pressure and feels like rest is always out of reach. People who may appear steady on the outside but feel frayed and fatigued on the inside. It's for those who feel like they're always pushing but are never quite catching up. To help make sense of what's happening, I'll introduce you to a simple but powerful model: The Mental Health Bucket Model.

In this model, your stress load is visualized as a bucket. Stressors are the inputs that pour into your bucket from the top—things like deadlines, emotional labor, unresolved conflict, personal loss, perfectionism, overscheduling, constant notifications, social media, and that internal voice that never stops criticizing. These inputs build up fast, even if you don't always notice them. The bucket also has drains—ways your system releases tension. These include sleep, movement, nourishing food, rest, joy, laughter, connection, therapy, mindfulness, and creativity. If these drains are intact and consistently maintained, your bucket can stay balanced. Even with high pressure, you won't overflow. But if the drains are blocked, or if the inputs come faster than they can be released, the system backs up—and that overflow is burnout.

No two people have the same bucket size, just as no two fingerprints are alike.

Each person also has their own bucket size—their individual capacity to carry stress before they hit their limit. Your capacity is shaped by many things: your genetics, medical conditions, hormone shifts, trauma history, social support, and even your past coping mechanisms.[16,17,18] Some of these factors you can influence; others you simply have to understand and work around. No two people have the same bucket size, just as no two fingerprints are alike. It's important not to compare yours to someone else's. Respecting your own limits is essential.

When too much pours in and not enough drains out—or if your bucket shrinks without your awareness—symptoms begin to surface. You may notice brain fog, forgetfulness, irritability, emotional numbness, anxiety, or a deep exhaustion that no amount of sleep seems to fix. Burnout doesn't wait for a dramatic breakdown to make itself known. It can appear slowly, and long before a crisis hits, the signs may already be there. The goal isn't to wait for that moment. The goal is to recognize what's happening and start clearing the water early.

This book was written to help you do just that. Not by offering motivational platitudes or impossible ideals, but by giving you grounded, research-based tools to reclaim your energy and clarity. By weaving together what's called the *biopsychosocial* influences on capacity (your bucket size), the daily pressures that pour in (your faucets), and the recovery systems that release tension (your drains), the model translates the science of stress and burnout into a framework that is simple enough to see, yet robust enough to act upon. You'll learn how to better understand your own capacity, identify the unseen inputs that are drowning you, and reestablish the rhythms that help your nervous system recover. You'll explore ways to open up the drains that support your well-being—like sleep, movement, mindfulness, and connection—and learn how to integrate small but powerful changes into your everyday life. The goal is not to withdraw from the people and responsibilities that matter to you but to stay engaged without losing yourself in the process.

This isn't a survival guide—it's a recovery map. *Burnout: Where the Head Goes, the Body Follows* is built on the belief that burnout isn't a personal failure. It's a signal. A call to shift from judgment to understanding, from collapse to recalibration. No matter how foggy or fractured things feel right now, you can find clarity again. And it begins not with fixing everything but with finding space. It starts with one breath, one shift, one moment of calm. Because when the head steadies, the body can follow—and healing begins.

1

The Dimensions of a Human

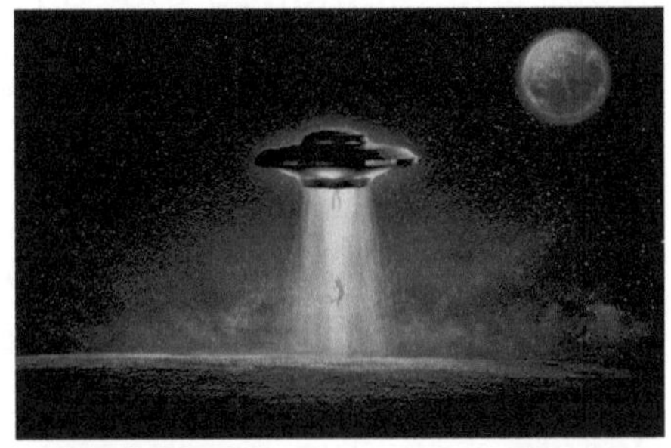

HERE'S A QUESTION worth sitting with for a moment—a rhetorical, perhaps even unanswerable one, but one that can be insightful: How would an alien interpret what it means to be human? The thought itself isn't just a curiosity. It offers a rare opportunity to step outside the assumptions, habits, and filters that shape how you view yourself. It's a chance to observe your existence from a fresh, unbiased lens, as if you were studying the human experience for the first time.

From the outside looking in, an alien would likely begin with the obvious. A human being, in its most visible form, is a complex biological structure made of flesh, bone, tissue, and a network of intricate systems.[1] There's the circulatory system carrying oxygen and nutrients, the nervous system transmitting signals and storing memories, and the digestive system breaking down fuel. Each system has its own function, all collaborating to sustain life. The body's needs are nonnegotiable. You breathe because you must. You eat because your cells demand it. You sleep because your brain depends on it. These are the raw mechanics of being alive—a physical machine that requires constant maintenance and care.

But the alien wouldn't stop there. It wouldn't take long before another layer became apparent. Imagine two humans with nearly identical bodies, of similar age, health, and environment. Yet one approaches life with calm, confidence, and joy, while the other feels overwhelmed, isolated, or lost. What explains the difference? This is where the mind enters the picture—the operator of the system.[2] Not just the brain as a physical organ, but the thoughts, emotions, perspectives, and memories that shape how a person experiences the world.[3] This is what is often referred to as one's mental wellness, mental health, or mindset.

One of the most important distinctions in this area comes from psychologist Carol Dweck's theory of fixed versus growth mindset.[4,5] A fixed mindset assumes that intelligence, abilities, or personality traits are largely unchangeable. People with this perspective often see setbacks as proof of inadequacy, making stress feel heavier and progress harder. By contrast, a growth mindset views challenges as opportunities to learn, adapt, and expand one's abilities. Instead of interpreting struggle as failure, it becomes a signal to persist. Research shows that individuals with a growth mindset recover from setbacks more quickly, display greater resilience, and are less likely to burn out under pressure. Cultivating this way of thinking doesn't eliminate stress, but it reframes it—transforming pressure from a sign of limitation into a chance for development.

Here is where most introspection tends to pause. You might focus on your thoughts, try to regulate your emotions, adopt healthier habits, or build psychological resilience. All of that is foundational. But there is more to you than body and mind. There is another dimension—one that may not show up on a scan or in a lab result, but that is just as real: the spirit, or soul. Science may not offer a neat definition for it, and there's no device to measure its presence. Yet you've likely felt its influence in your own life. Consider what happens at the moment of death. One moment a person is breathing, thinking, and expressing. The next, the body is still there—but something vital is gone. Something unseen. For many, that absence speaks volumes.

Whether or not you use the word *soul*, you've probably sensed there's something more to your being than biology and cognition. A much more sophisticated discussion from a religious standpoint can be held to further understand, analyze, and reach spiritual elevation, which is beyond the scope of this book. However, it is important to acknowledge the extraordinary power this layer of you holds. It's where you search for meaning, connection, and purpose. It's where awe lives, and where peace takes root. When you nurture this layer, life doesn't just become bearable—it becomes deeply fulfilling. Think of it this way: Mental health may be the steady fuel that keeps your life running, but spiritual insight is rocket fuel. It allows you to rise above the noise, transcend the chaos, and touch something bigger than yourself.

Now imagine your alien observer noticing all three layers: your body, your mind, and your soul. Each one tells part of the story, but only together do they offer a complete picture of what it means to be you. That's the real invitation here—to start seeing yourself from that broader perspective. To understand your life not as a series of tasks or reactions, but as a system—one that needs care, attention, and balance across all dimensions.

The pressures of modern life are unlikely to stop anytime soon. Work demands, financial stress, relationship struggles, and personal expectations will continue to rise and fall in waves. But what you can change is how you manage them: how you care for your inputs, how you respond to overload, how you protect your energy, and where you look for meaning when everything feels like too much.

This book offers you a model to help map that process—a simple framework that captures how stress, emotion, and recovery flow through your internal systems. It's designed to help you visualize how life's pressures affect your mental state and how to restore your balance. But before diving into that, take a moment to zoom out. Reflect on your own layers. Your body, yes—but also your thoughts, your feelings, your beliefs, your soul. How well are these dimensions integrated into your daily life? Which ones have been neglected? Which ones are quietly asking for your attention?

You don't need to chase perfection. Start by chasing awareness. Understanding yourself from the outside in—and the inside out—gives you something more powerful than any quick fix: It gives you the ability to see clearly. From that clarity, balance becomes possible. Healing becomes real. And growth becomes inevitable. That's where your journey continues.

2

The Mass Balance Equation

Input - Output = Accumulation

NOW IMAGINE YOUR alien observer narrowing their focus—not on the broad human experience, but on the intricate mechanics beneath the surface of your skin. Their attention shifts to how your physical form operates—how the body keeps itself alive through complex, interdependent systems. During my own journey—first as a biomedical engineer, then as a physician—I spent years immersed in this very architecture. In engineering, I learned to see the body as a system: inputs, outputs, feedback loops, and error tolerances.[1] In medicine, I added flesh to that framework—countless hours studying anatomy, long days in dissection labs, and sleepless nights on clinical rotations. With every layer I peeled back, the same truth emerged: The human body is not a collection of parts. It is a living system—an orchestra of interdependent subsystems designed to maintain one critical goal: equilibrium.

The human body is a living system—an orchestra of interdependent subsystems designed to maintain one critical goal: equilibrium.

Your cardiovascular, digestive, pulmonary, nervous, renal, and skeletal systems may each have distinct roles, but none operates in isolation. Each system continuously exchanges signals, energy, and resources with the others, working to preserve your internal stability—what we refer to in both medicine and engineering as *homeostasis*. Unlike moods or thoughts, these systems are tangible. You can image a heart, trace a nerve, observe a muscle contract. They're measurable, and because of that, medicine has studied them rigorously for centuries. Yet beneath the surface-level anatomy and lab values lies something I first encountered not in a hospital but in my engineering coursework: the concept of mass balance.

At its core, mass balance is deceptively simple. Any system, biological or mechanical, operates by the same fundamental equation: What enters (inputs) minus what leaves (outputs) equals what accumulates.[2] But within this simplicity lies a powerful lens to understand both our bodies and our broader human experience.

Take your lungs, for example. Air flows in, oxygen is absorbed, and carbon dioxide is expelled. If that balance is disrupted—by inflammation, infection, or pollution—waste accumulates, and the system becomes inefficient. Breathing becomes labored. The imbalance reveals itself. Let's consider the heart: Blood enters, rich with oxygen and nutrients, and is pumped outward to nourish every cell. But if there's a blockage or dysfunction—be it structural, electrical, or pressure-related—the flow breaks down and the system starts to fail. Your kidneys, liver, and digestive tract all operate on this same principle of constantly receiving, filtering, converting, and releasing. If the inputs are overwhelming, or the outputs are impaired, accumulation builds—and systems suffer.

However, mass balance doesn't just apply to organs. It governs your entire life. Every day you're taking in inputs—not just food and oxygen, but emotional, psychological, and informational loads. The emails, the deadlines, the expectations, the news, the unresolved conversations, the chronic worry—these all pour into your system. They are real inputs, even if invisible. And then there's your output—your way of processing, releasing, expressing. Do you move your body? Talk things out? Sleep well? Create space to decompress? Or are you silently absorbing more than you're releasing, allowing stress to collect like plaque in an artery?

When the balance tips—when inputs exceed outputs over time—you begin to feel it. Accumulated strain appears as physical tension, restlessness, fatigue, mood swings, sleeplessness, or even numbness. You may not recognize how much you've internalized until your system reaches its threshold. This slow accumulation is often how burnout begins. Not with a dramatic event, but with the quiet stacking of unmet demands, unattended stress, and delayed recovery. Small mismatches—between what life requires and what you can sustainably deliver—compound into chronic overload.

Through the lens of engineering, this imbalance is measurable. Through the lens of medicine, it is diagnosable. But through the lens of your own life, it is deeply personal. And the moment you begin seeing your experience in terms of mass balance, you gain something essential: clarity. You begin recognizing where your major inputs come from, where your outputs are insufficient, and where silent accumulation is building up. You're no longer at the mercy of burnout; you start becoming a systems operator.

This awareness is not about eliminating stress altogether. In fact, some level of stress—like voltage in a circuit or tension in a muscle—is necessary for function. But systems, whether engineered or biological, require periodic recalibration. They need time to recover, clear buildup, and restore baseline function. Your mind and body are no exception.

In the next chapter, you'll apply this mass balance framework directly to your mental health. We'll map your emotional and cognitive inputs, identify the strength of your outputs, and make the invisible visible—so you can take back control of the load you're carrying.

Before you move on, take a moment to pause. You are now the system under observation. Not from a distance, and not from another planet, but from within. Your goal isn't to engineer a perfect self overnight. It's to start noticing the flow—what comes in, what goes out, and what lingers. Once you do, you can start designing your life not just for survival but for balance. And, eventually, for resilience.

3

Mental Health Features – The "Bucket" Model

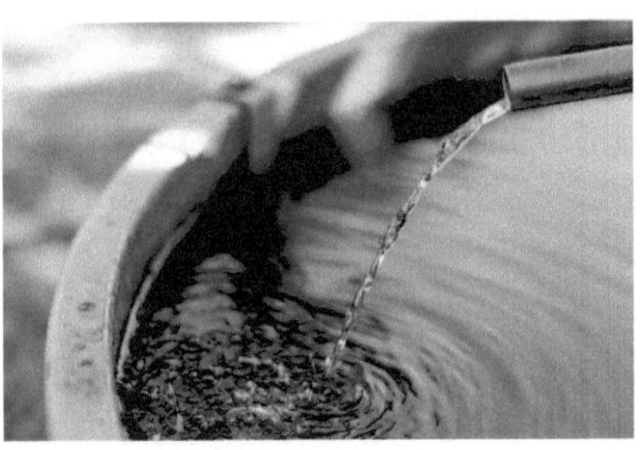

YOUR MENTAL HEALTH system, like any other system, has inputs, outputs, and accumulation. But unlike the body's visible systems, this domain operates beneath the surface. You can't see the slow buildup until it starts to overflow. And when it does, one of the most common outcomes is something you may know too well: burnout.

> **Your mental health system, like any other system, has inputs, outputs, and accumulation.**

Burnout isn't simply about being tired or overwhelmed after a long week. You've felt ordinary exhaustion before, and you've recovered from it with some rest. This is different. Burnout is a slow, progressive erosion of your emotional and psychological resources. It shows up as emotional exhaustion that doesn't fade, a growing detachment from work or people you care about, and a quiet but nagging sense that your efforts aren't making a difference.[1]

You feel like you're running on empty, even though you're still trying just as hard as you always have. At some point, you begin to wonder: How did it get like this?

The truth is, it rarely happens in a single moment. It builds over time, one drop at a time. To understand how, imagine for a moment that you're carrying an internal bucket—a simple but powerful way to visualize your mental health. This bucket represents your capacity to handle stress and to carry the pressures and responsibilities that life hands you. Your bucket has a certain size. That size isn't random; it's shaped by your genetics, your upbringing, your personal history, and your life experiences.[2,3,4] Some people naturally have larger buckets, able to absorb a great deal before reaching their limit. Others have smaller ones, filling more quickly under similar pressures. Even two people growing up in the same household can carry buckets of entirely different shapes and sizes.

Now think about what fills that bucket. Each stressor you encounter is like a faucet turned on above it. Some faucets release a steady, small stream—maybe the daily grind of work or parenting. Others can suddenly blast open—a financial crisis, a major health scare, a relationship breakdown. You may even carry faucets you barely notice: unresolved childhood wounds, perfectionistic tendencies, or a constant internal pressure to succeed. The water from each faucet adds up. As it pours in, the level rises. At first, your bucket manages just fine. You absorb the flow, adjust, and keep moving forward. But over time, as more faucets stay open or new ones appear, the level creeps higher. Eventually, it reaches the brim.

At that point, it doesn't take much to send the water spilling over. A critical email, a fight with a loved one, a small setback—something that might seem insignificant to others—becomes the drop that breaks the surface. What they see as an overreaction is really the moment your system overflows. The burnout isn't about that one drop. It's about everything that came before it. If an outside observer—like that curious alien from earlier—were to watch you in that moment, they might struggle to understand why something so minor would provoke such a strong reaction. But the reason is simple: When a bucket is full, even a drop can trigger a crisis.

You've probably seen people carry full buckets without realizing it. Perhaps you've done it yourself. You push through, assuming that this is just how life is supposed to feel. You tell yourself you should be able to handle it. And because burnout often builds quietly, you don't always recognize how close you are to the edge until you're already there. What matters now is not judgment but awareness. Because once you see your life in terms of the Mental Health Bucket Model, you also see that burnout is not a personal weakness. It's not about lacking willpower or failing to "tough it out." It's simply an imbalance—a system pushed beyond its limits. And that means it can be corrected.

There are three primary ways to regain control. First, you can reduce the inflow. You can turn down the faucets by setting boundaries, saying no to additional responsibilities, resolving long-standing conflicts, or reevaluating obligations that no longer serve you. Every bit of stress you reduce lowers the water level. Second, you can drain the bucket. You create outlets to release pressure. This might include rest, exercise, therapy, hobbies, creative outlets, spiritual practices, or simply allowing yourself space to recover. Each of these helps drain accumulated stress and restore balance. Third, you can expand the bucket. Over time, you can build greater capacity. This might happen through personal growth, stronger coping skills, supportive relationships, or professional guidance. Expanding your bucket means you can handle greater challenges without overflowing as easily.

These aren't abstract concepts. They are real strategies you can apply to your life, starting exactly where you are. The goal is not to empty your bucket but to prevent it from constantly teetering on the edge. In the chapters ahead, you'll dive deeper into how this model works in practice. You'll map your own inputs, explore your drains, and identify where accumulation may be quietly taking place. By making these invisible processes visible, you'll give yourself the tools to intervene early—before burnout takes hold—or to recover if it already has. This isn't just a theoretical exercise. This is your system. And now you're beginning to see it clearly.

4

The Bucket Size

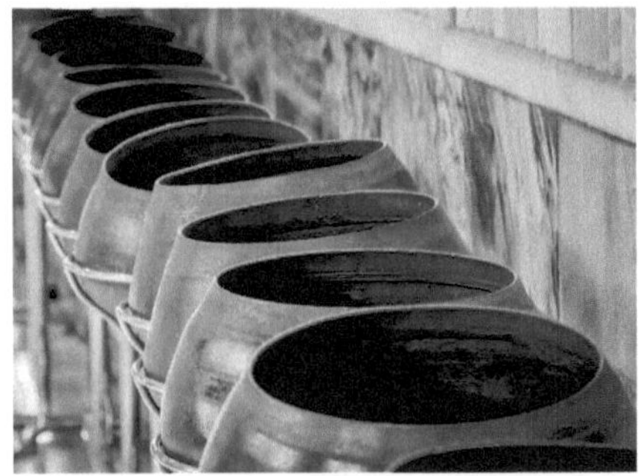

BEFORE DIVING INTO the many faucets that pour stress into your bucket or the drains that help relieve the pressure, it's worth pausing to examine the bucket itself—specifically, its size. This isn't just an academic exercise. The size of your bucket quietly shapes how you experience stress, how easily you reach your breaking point, and how much room you have to absorb life's inevitable challenges. And out of all the moving parts in this system, your bucket size is the one factor you control the least, and the one that likely takes the longest to adjust.

Your default capacity isn't something you chose. You didn't design it or select it like an item off a menu. Instead, it has been shaped over years—by forces both within and outside of you. In the mental health world, these forces are often described as *biopsychosocial factors*.[1,2] It's a long word for something deeply personal: your biology, your psychology, and your social environment—all working together to define your resilience and vulnerability.

It helps to think of yourself like a plant growing in a garden. Some plants are born with ideal conditions—rich soil, steady sunshine, clean water. Others have grown in rocky soil, under constant shade, or in unpredictable climates. In this analogy, your biopsychosocial factors are the soil, water, and sunlight that have surrounded you from the beginning. None of this was your choice, but all of it has quietly shaped how your plant has grown—and how sturdy or fragile it may feel today.

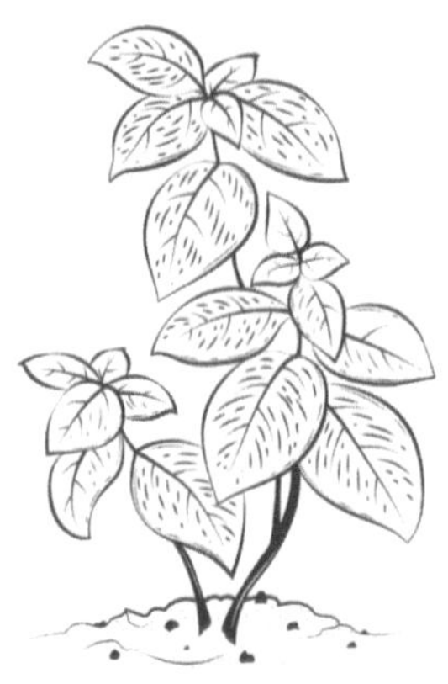

It helps to think of yourself like a plant growing in a garden—your biopsychosocial factors are the soil, water, and sunlight that have surrounded you from the beginning.

Start with the seed itself. This represents your genetics—your DNA, your inherited temperament, the raw material you were born with. These genetics quietly influence how your brain responds to stress, how quickly you recover from adversity, and how sensitive you are to emotional strain.[3,4] Some people naturally carry a baseline of emotional steadiness, while others are wired for heightened sensitivity, reactivity, or worry. Neither is right or wrong—they simply are.

But no seed grows in isolation. The soil it lands in matters deeply. This is where your early life environment comes into play—the parenting you received, the stability of your home, your family's financial security, exposure to safety or trauma, access to education and healthcare, and the cultural messages you absorbed along the way. Many of these factors are now referred to as *social determinants of health*.[5,6,7] A seed in nutrient-rich soil has a very different experience than one planted in dry, rocky ground. The more supportive and stable your environment, the stronger your roots likely became. The more stressful or chaotic your early years, the more fragile those roots may feel now.

Sunlight and water will continue to nurture or stress the plant over time. This includes your ongoing life circumstances—your friendships, work environment, financial pressures, health challenges, and the presence or absence of a support network.[8,9] Even as an adult, the conditions you live in continue to shape the resilience of your bucket.

And then there are the storms—those unexpected events that hit without warning. A sudden illness, the loss of a loved one, a traumatic event, a financial collapse. Some people weather these storms with relatively little damage, while others are deeply affected.[10,11] Often it's not the storm itself but the condition of the plant beforehand that determines how much harm is done.

When you step back and consider your own life through this lens, you begin to see why your bucket may feel bigger or smaller than someone else's. Two people may face the same stressor but experience it very differently—not because one is stronger or weaker, but because each has been shaped by a different combination of soil, seed, sunlight, and storms.

Understanding your bucket size isn't about making excuses or assigning blame. It's about seeing yourself clearly—accepting the hand you've been dealt so you can work with it rather than fight against it. If your bucket feels small, that's not a moral failing. It simply means you may need to be more intentional about managing stress, setting boundaries, and building support systems. If your bucket feels larger, you may have more room to take on challenges, but that doesn't make you invincible.

And even though you can't fully control your bucket size, you can still influence it. Over time—with the right tools, therapy, habits, and supportive relationships—it's possible to strengthen your resilience, build new coping skills, and expand your capacity.[12,13,14] The soil may have been rocky at the start, but with care and attention, new nutrients can be added. The plant can still grow stronger.

Before you move forward to explore the specific stressors that pour into your bucket—or the drains that help release pressure—it's helpful to understand some of the key elements that influence your capacity. In the coming chapters, we will explore your genetic vulnerabilities and inherited traits; your innate temperament and personality style; chronic health conditions that may add strain; the impact of socioeconomic pressures and access to resources; your family dynamics and early childhood experiences; the lingering effects of trauma or loss; and underlying biological or neurological factors that affect emotional processing.

Each of these plays a role in defining how full your bucket gets and how quickly it reaches overflow. You don't have to master them all right now. But simply recognizing that these forces exist helps you approach yourself with more compassion—and arms you with insight as you begin to build strategies that fit your life, not someone else's. Now it's time to start unpacking these pieces one by one—beginning with your genetic wiring, and how it quietly shapes your resilience every single day.

4.1 Genetic Vulnerability

As science has advanced, so has the understanding of how genetics shape our mental health. The breakthroughs from the Human Genome Project opened an entirely new window into how our DNA influences not only physical conditions but also our emotional well-being.[15] This growing knowledge offers important clues about why you might respond to stress the way you do.

When I sit with patients, one of the most valuable tools I use is a simple conversation about family history. It's not just about listing illnesses; it's about identifying patterns that reveal genetic tendencies passed down across generations. Mental health conditions like autism spectrum disorder, bipolar disorder, major depression, and schizophrenia often show strong genetic links.[16] If these conditions exist within your family tree, they quietly lower your personal threshold for stress tolerance and emotional resilience.

But having a genetic vulnerability doesn't mean you are destined to develop one of these disorders. Your DNA doesn't write an unchangeable script—it simply creates a predisposition.[17] Think of it as a lowered starting point on your stress scale. For someone else, it might take years of overwhelming pressure to reach a breaking point. For you, that threshold may be closer, requiring fewer stressors to tip the balance.

This knowledge isn't meant to instill fear. It's meant to offer clarity. The better you understand your own genetic wiring, the more intentionally you can protect your mental health. You may need to be more proactive about setting boundaries, creating recovery routines, and seeking support before small stressors accumulate into something heavier. You aren't fragile—but you may be finely tuned.

Seeing your genetics as one piece of your bucket helps you step into ownership rather than helplessness. It explains some of the invisible weight you may carry and reminds you of why personalized strategies matter so much. Your path toward resilience won't look like anyone else's, because your internal wiring is uniquely yours.

As you continue to explore the rest of the biopsychosocial factors, you'll begin to see the full landscape of what fills and shapes your bucket. And with that understanding comes the power to manage it—carefully, deliberately, and in a way that honors who you are.

4.2 Temperament

Beyond your genetic blueprint, another piece quietly shapes the size of your bucket: your temperament. Genetics may set the foundation, but temperament shows how you first began to meet the world, even in your earliest days.

You've likely noticed certain patterns in how you respond to stress or stimulation—patterns that have been with you for as long as you can remember. That's temperament at work. The American Psychological Association describes it as "the basic foundation of personality, usually assumed to be biologically determined and present early in life, including such characteristics as energy level, emotional responsiveness, demeanor, mood, response tempo, behavioral inhibition, and willingness to explore."[18]

In simpler terms, it's the earliest expression of your psychological identity—like the first shoot emerging from the soil. This shoot may reach upward with confidence or stay closer to the ground, cautious and observant. From the very beginning, your temperament has shaped whether you lean toward curiosity or caution, whether you respond calmly or with heightened emotion, whether you seek novelty or prefer predictability.[19]

Temperament is the earliest expression of your psychological identity—like the first shoot emerging from the soil.

As life unfolds, these early tendencies often remain, quietly influencing how you experience the world.[20] Maybe transitions have always felt unsettling to you, while others seem to embrace them with ease. Maybe you find yourself feeling deeply affected by emotions that others seem able to shrug off. These aren't flaws. They're reflections of how you're naturally wired.

Unfortunately, it's easy to dismiss these patterns once you reach adulthood, as if childhood tendencies no longer matter. But those early imprints continue to affect how much stress your bucket can hold today. When certain situations feel heavier or recovery from setbacks seems harder, your temperament often holds part of the explanation.

Recognizing your temperament allows you to approach stress and burnout from a place of compassion, not self-criticism. You're not failing because something feels hard—you're responding according to your design. And by understanding that design, you gain the ability to build coping strategies that fit who you are, instead of forcing yourself into approaches that work better for someone else.

With this piece in place, you can start to see the bigger picture of your unique capacity. Next, it's time to explore how chronic medical conditions can further shape—and sometimes limit—the size of your bucket.

4.3 Chronic Medical Conditions

Another layer shaping the size of your mental health bucket comes from chronic medical conditions. While temperament reflects how you're internally wired, chronic illness introduces persistent, often invisible stressors that steadily erode resilience over time.

The connection between chronic physical illness and mental health isn't just a loose association—it's deeply intertwined. The National Institute of Mental Health (NIMH) highlights a long list of conditions linked to higher rates of anxiety and depression: Alzheimer's disease, autoimmune disorders, cancer, coronary heart disease, diabetes, epilepsy, HIV/AIDS, hypothyroidism, Parkinson's disease, and stroke.[21] Living with any of these conditions demands constant adaptation. Each symptom, appointment, or side effect quietly adds weight to your mental load. The stress is never purely physical. It seeps into emotions, relationships, and sense of self, often in ways that others may not fully see or understand.

Among these, chronic pain stands out as especially debilitating. Pain that lingers long after the body should have healed—whether from back injuries, arthritis, migraines, cancer treatments, or nerve damage—acts like a slow, constant erosion into the bucket. It doesn't just interfere with daily routines; it chips away at energy, patience, and optimism.[22,23] Many describe a painful triad that clinicians sometimes call the *terrible triad*: sleeplessness, sadness, and persistent discomfort.[24] Over time, this combination can wear down even the strongest mental defenses.

When pain or illness becomes part of daily life, irritability, isolation, and hopelessness often follow. The bucket fills faster, sometimes with little warning. And while others may assume life appears stable from the outside, the internal struggle tells a very different story.

But even here, there's space for hope. Many chronic conditions—especially chronic pain—respond not only to medical treatments but also to psychological approaches. *Pain psychology* offers tools like cognitive reframing, behavioral therapy, coping strategies, and emotional support, helping reduce the emotional weight of living with ongoing health challenges.[25]

By acknowledging the role of chronic medical conditions, it becomes easier to understand why some buckets feel heavier even during ordinary life circumstances. It isn't weakness—it's accumulation. Each person carries a load shaped not only by stressors but by the quiet, enduring presence of their physical health.

Next, it's time to explore how socioeconomic status adds yet another layer to this equation, shaping access to resources, stability, and recovery.

Case Example:

Rob had lived with chronic back pain since his early 30s. For years, it had been manageable—occasional flare-ups after long hours or strenuous days. But more recently, the pain had become persistent. Even gentle activities like walking or stretching triggered discomfort. Determined to stay active, John pushed through, but his body pushed back. Every step became a negotiation. With movement now tied to discomfort, he started withdrawing. He declined weekend outings, skipped his usual errands, and slowly retreated from the small joys that once anchored his days. His mood dipped. Irritability crept in. He gained weight, which only worsened the pain, creating a loop that felt harder to escape by the week. At the urging of a longtime friend, John visited his primary care provider. After basic labs and imaging, he was referred to pain management and physical therapy. That's where he was introduced to aquatic exercises—movements in water that took pressure off his spine and joints. It wasn't a cure, but it was a turning point. Bit by bit, he started feeling stronger. He could move without bracing for pain. His energy returned. He smiled more. And most importantly, he began to understand something he hadn't seen before: that his physical pain wasn't just limiting his body—it had been quietly reshaping his mental health. Rob's breakthrough wasn't just about treatment. It was about recognition. By acknowledging the full impact of his condition—physically and emotionally—he gained tools, options, and a renewed sense of agency. His pain didn't vanish, but it no longer defined him. Now he moves through life with more clarity, more strength, and a deeper respect for the way the body and mind speak to one another—always.

4.4 Socioeconomic Status

Socioeconomic status quietly shapes the size of your mental health bucket in ways that are often easy to overlook, but impossible to escape. It threads through the fabric of everyday life, influencing both the stress you absorb and the resources available to release it. This interplay is best understood within the broader concept of social determinants of health—the conditions in which people are born, grow, live, work, and age.[26] These determinants aren't just distant policy issues; they are deeply personal realities. Housing stability, employment opportunities, education access, food security, neighborhood safety, and reliable transportation—all of these either help widen your bucket or constrict it.

To see how this unfolds in human terms, consider Maslow's Hierarchy of Needs. In 1943, psychologist Abraham Maslow proposed a model in his paper *A Theory of Human Motivation*, describing a progression of needs beginning with the most fundamental: physiological stability and safety.[27] Food, water, shelter, and financial security form the base. Only when these foundational needs are consistently met can someone begin to focus on higher goals—relationships, confidence, creativity, and self-actualization. But real life rarely climbs this ladder in a straight line. A job loss, rent spike, illness, or car breakdown can snap focus back to survival. When basic needs are on shaky ground, emotional regulation and long-term planning take a back seat. Anxiety becomes chronic. The nervous system stays on alert. The margin for error disappears.

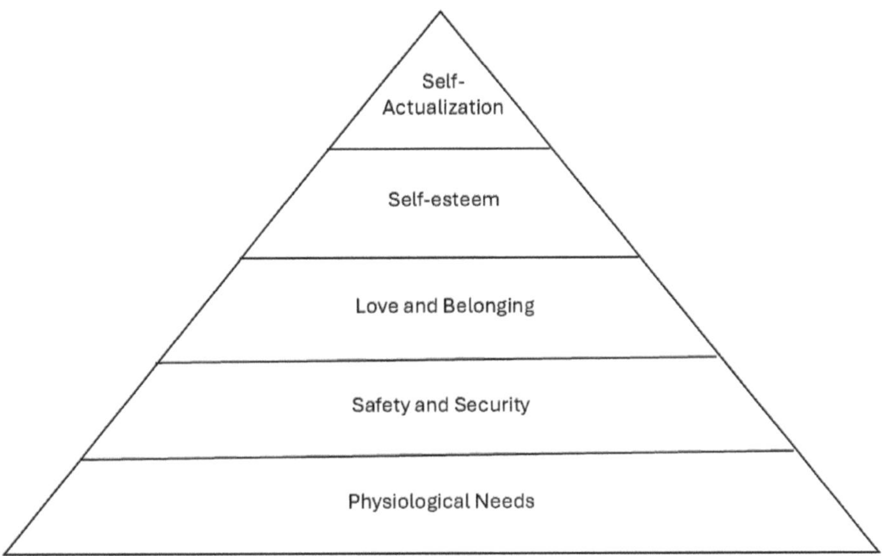

This isn't speculation—it's backed by contemporary evidence. A global study examining data from 201 countries between 1970 and 2020 showed a robust positive association between unemployment and a variety of mental disorders, including anxiety and depression.[28] Lower-income populations consistently face higher rates of psychological distress—not because of personal weakness, but due to sustained exposure to economic instability, limited resources, and harsher environments. Under these conditions, your mental health bucket doesn't just fill faster—it likely starts smaller. And that smaller capacity makes every additional stressor feel disproportionately heavy.

Understanding the link between social determinants and mental health helps reframe the conversation. It offers a more compassionate lens. Struggling isn't a sign of personal inadequacy—it's often the result of prolonged tension inside systems that were never built for equity. When someone is worried about making rent, affording medications, or keeping food on the table, it makes sense that energy for growth, reflection, or emotional processing feels out of reach. The constant push to survive takes a toll on emotional bandwidth.

Recognizing these structural factors can be empowering. It shifts blame from internal character to external context and invites more realistic, sustainable strategies for healing. It also opens the door to external support—whether that's accessing local community programs, seeking financial counseling, connecting with housing assistance services, or finding therapy that acknowledges cultural and economic barriers. These are not luxuries; they are lifelines for people navigating a system that is often unforgiving.

There's still another layer influencing the size of the bucket: the emotional tone of the family environment and the imprints left by early caregiving relationships. These roots run deep, and they shape how you absorb, carry, and respond to stress. The next part of the journey begins there.

4.5 Family Dynamic

Another element involved in shaping mental health capacity—sometimes more powerfully than any other—is the family dynamic. Family is the first school we attend, silently teaching us how to feel, connect, and cope with the world. This influence doesn't wait until birth to begin. Long before a child takes their first breath, development is already in motion. While the fetus receives physical nourishment through the umbilical cord, it is also shaped by the mother's habits, emotions, and environment.[29] Exposure to substances such as alcohol, nicotine, or drugs during pregnancy can leave lasting effects on the developing brain and body.[30] Even maternal stress, through elevated levels of stress hormones like cortisol, can influence how the baby's stress regulation system is wired.[31]

Family is the first school we attend.

After birth, learning unfolds primarily through connection, which is referred to as *attachment theory*.[32] Long before children speak, they become fluent in the nonverbal language of relationships. They read facial expressions, body language, tone of voice, and emotional cues. From this, they learn what safety feels like, what comfort looks like, and how emotions are managed. They observe and internalize how parents and caregivers respond to conflict, sadness, disappointment, and joy. Children mirror what they see. Every reaction—every reward, punishment, or moment of silence—becomes part of the internal blueprint they carry into adulthood. These patterns shape how they handle stress, form relationships, and regulate their emotions. This foundational learning often occurs quietly, without instruction, and usually without conscious awareness.

In this way, the family truly becomes the first classroom. Developmental psychologist Erik Erikson mapped this progression through his model of psychosocial development, which outlines eight critical life stages, each marked by a core emotional task.[33] In infancy, the task is trust versus mistrust, where the consistency and warmth of a caregiver determine whether the world feels safe. During early childhood, autonomy versus shame and doubt comes into play, with children building confidence through supportive independence or developing shame under excessive control. The preschool years bring initiative versus guilt, where encouragement fosters a sense of capability and criticism breeds guilt. In school-age years, children navigate industry versus inferiority, with success in school and social settings creating pride, and failure or comparison leading to inadequacy.

As adolescence unfolds, the task becomes identity versus role confusion, where youth explore their beliefs, values, and self-concept. Support fosters a confident identity, while instability leads to confusion. In young adulthood, intimacy versus isolation centers around emotional closeness and vulnerability; unresolved fears here often create loneliness. Middle adulthood brings the stage of generativity versus stagnation, as individuals seek to contribute to society and those around them. Lack of purpose here breeds stagnation. Finally, in late adulthood, individuals face ego integrity versus despair, reflecting on life with either a sense of fulfillment or regret.

Each of these stages presents both an opportunity and a risk. The family's role—whether as a stabilizing presence or a source of stress—remains pivotal at every phase. The impact of parents, caregivers, and siblings leaves marks both visible and subtle, many of which persist for decades. When families provide emotional safety, consistency, and structure, mental health capacity grows. These environments support the development of healthy coping mechanisms, emotional regulation, and self-esteem. In contrast, when family dynamics are characterized by chaos, criticism, neglect, or abuse, emotional resilience is compromised. The mental health bucket becomes smaller and fills more quickly with stress.

Understanding the role of family dynamics is not about assigning blame—it's about cultivating awareness. Recognizing how early relationships shaped your emotional responses allows for deeper insight. You may begin to understand why certain situations trigger disproportionate stress, why emotional patterns repeat in your relationships, or why some feelings linger longer than expected. With that understanding, you can begin to create space for healing. And from here, the journey turns toward another foundational force that often overlaps with family life and leaves a lasting imprint: trauma.

Stage	Age Range	Core Conflict	Positive Outcome	Negative Outcome
Infancy	0–1 year	Trust vs. Mistrust	Develops a sense of trust in the world through consistent care	Develops mistrust and fear if care is inconsistent or neglectful
Early Childhood	1–3 years	Autonomy vs. Shame and Doubt	Gains confidence and independence through support	Develops shame or doubt due to excessive control or criticism
Preschool	3–5 years	Initiative vs. Guilt	Learns initiative through encouragement and exploration	Develops guilt if overly restricted or criticized
School Age	6–12 years	Industry vs. Inferiority	Builds pride and competence through school and social success	Feels inferior from repeated failure or comparison
Adolescence	12–18 years	Identity vs. Role Confusion	Forms a confident and stable self-identity through exploration	Experiences confusion or instability about self and life direction
Young Adulthood	18–40 years	Intimacy vs. Isolation	Forms deep emotional connections and close relationships	Suffers loneliness and isolation from fear of vulnerability
Middle Adulthood	40–65 years	Generativity vs. Stagnation	Finds purpose in contributing to others and society	Feels stuck or unproductive if unable to find meaningful engagement
Late Adulthood	65+ years	Ego Integrity vs. Despair	Reflects on life with fulfillment and wisdom	Experiences regret, bitterness, or despair over past life choices

4.6 Trauma

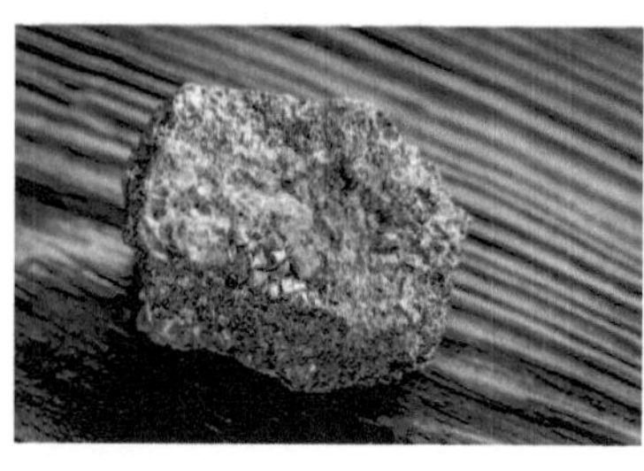

Now comes one of the most delicate, deeply personal, and often life-shaping influences on mental wellness: trauma. Within the Mental Health Bucket Model, trauma holds a particular significance. Trauma sits in the bucket like a rock, taking up space and adding more weight, until one takes steps to chisel it down. That rock doesn't need to spill over to be significant; its very presence reduces how much more the bucket can hold. Once trauma is lodged in your system, it limits your available capacity for everything else that life brings your way.

Trauma sits in the bucket like a rock, taking up space and adding more weight, until one takes steps to chisel it down.

Trauma takes many forms. The Substance Abuse and Mental Health Services Administration (SAMHSA), in *TIP 57: Trauma-Informed Care in Behavioral Health Services*, defines trauma as "an event, series of events, or set of circumstances that is experienced by an individual as physically or emotionally harmful or life threatening and that has lasting adverse effects on the individual's functioning and mental, physical, social, emotional, or spiritual well-being."[34] Trauma reaches far into a person's relationships, decisions, sense of self-worth, and emotional resilience—often long after the original event has ended.

To better understand trauma, it can help to think of it in three general categories. Simple acute trauma refers to a single distressing event that may cause fear or shock but does not linger for years. Chronic stress, on the other hand, is the slow, steady drip of ongoing hardship—perhaps a toxic relationship, persistent work pressure, or long-term financial instability. Traumatic stress refers to the most intense, life-altering experiences such as abuse, war, serious accidents, or profound loss. These typically affect every aspect of life and often require professional support to navigate.

To visualize the difference, imagine dropping objects into a calm lake. A single pebble might create a ripple—that's simple acute trauma. Chronic stress tosses pebble after pebble, disturbing the water repeatedly. But traumatic stress is the boulder. It sends waves crashing over the shoreline, shifting the entire system. Often the size of the impact isn't obvious from the surface, but its consequences are lasting.

How trauma manifests depends on more than just the nature of the event. It's also shaped by your age at the time, your support system, your coping strategies, your cultural lens, and the meaning you attach to what happened.[35] Two people can endure the same external experience but process it very differently. However, certain patterns of reactions are observed when one experiences significant trauma.[36,37,38] The early signs may include emotional confusion, sadness, numbness, anxiety, or agitation. Physically, it may show up as fatigue, hyperarousal, or a sense of disconnection from your surroundings. Over time, secondary symptoms can emerge: emotional distress that doesn't resolve, flashbacks, nightmares, insomnia, chronic hypervigilance, avoidance of triggers, or a persistent sense that the world is no longer safe. Trauma also increases the risk for depression and anxiety disorders.

Sometimes these reactions lie dormant for months or years before something triggers them—a smell, a song, a place. The body remembers, even if the conscious mind has tried to forget. But there is good news: The majority of people—nearly 80 percent—experience substantial recovery within a year, especially when supported by appropriate care and community. Healing may not erase the event, but it restores agency. It brings back your ability to feel joy, form secure relationships, sustain self-worth, and meet life's responsibilities.

Still, trauma often leaves behind a fingerprint in the form of deep-seated beliefs that can distort your internal world. Psychologist Aaron Beck's Cognitive Triad offers a useful lens for this. It refers to negative beliefs about yourself (*I'm broken*), about others and the world (*People can't be trusted*), and about the future (*Things will never get better*). These beliefs don't just remain idle—they shape how you view new experiences. They may lead to unhealthy coping behaviors such as substance use, compulsive habits, emotional withdrawal, or self-sabotage.

Fortunately, trauma is not a life sentence. Its weight can lessen, its grip can loosen, and its presence in your bucket can shrink. Therapy helps in this process. Whether through mindfulness, cognitive restructuring, trauma-focused modalities like EMDR, prolonged exposure, or somatic-based treatments, healing becomes a process of chipping away at the rock in the bucket, gradually freeing space for resilience to return.[39]

The aim of trauma-informed care is not merely to reduce symptoms but to create safety—a space where vulnerability is honored, not judged, and where emotional repair becomes not just possible but expected. In the context of the Mental Health Bucket Model, trauma is not just another form of stress that comes and goes. It's a presence that fills space until it's fully addressed. The larger the rock, the less room you have to handle everyday stress. But through sustained healing, that rock gets smaller, and your bucket's capacity to carry life improves.

As we continue forward, there's one more layer to examine—one that is often overlooked but critical in shaping mental resilience: the role of biological imbalances. These subtle physiological shifts can silently strain your mental health long before their presence is felt. Next, we'll explore how these forces might be shrinking your bucket without your awareness—and what to do about it.

Case Example:

Samantha had always sensed that her early years shaped the way she moved through the world. A childhood marked by emotional neglect and abuse left her cautious—guarded in new environments, slow to trust, and constantly on alert, even when things were calm. On the outside, her life looked stable: a long-term job, a supportive husband, and a close-knit circle of trusted friends. But internally, she felt constrained—held back by patterns she couldn't fully name. When she finally opened up to her primary care doctor, she was referred to trauma-focused therapy. The first few sessions were raw. Old memories surfaced, stirring emotions she had buried for decades. But her therapist helped her move through them with care—gently untangling her story without retraumatizing her in the process. Over time, something shifted. Samantha started to feel lighter, not because the past disappeared, but because it no longer carried the same weight. She found herself laughing more, accepting social invitations, and speaking up in meetings without the usual self-doubt. Confidence emerged not in dramatic changes, but in quiet, steady moments of presence. Her trauma didn't vanish—but it stopped dictating the terms of her life. With consistent support and her own deep courage, Samantha began reclaiming her narrative, one safe step at a time.

4.7 Biological Deficiencies

Now that you've unpacked the emotional weight of trauma, it's time to turn to something less visible—something that might not come with memories or scars, but that still has a major impact on how much stress you can carry: biological deficiencies. These imbalances might not be immediately noticeable, but they can slowly shrink your capacity for resilience, making everyday challenges feel heavier than they should. Unlike emotional or social factors, biological deficiencies often go unnoticed because they don't come with dramatic warning signs. Instead, they may appear as persistent fatigue, low mood, difficulty concentrating, irritability, or a subtle sense that something just feels "off."

The good news is that most of these deficiencies are both measurable and treatable. A simple blood test can uncover a lot and, once identified, these imbalances can often be corrected with the help of a healthcare provider. Think of them as silent cracks in your mental health bucket. They may not be the cause of an immediate overflow, but they weaken the overall structure, causing you to leak energy and clarity without understanding why.

Some of the most common biological contributors to mental health include vitamin D, folic acid (vitamin B9), vitamin B12, and thyroid function.[40,41,42] Vitamin D, often called the "sunshine vitamin," plays a significant role in neurotransmitter activity and immune function—both of which affect mood. Low levels are associated with depression, irritability, and fatigue. Folic acid is essential for DNA production and the synthesis of neurotransmitters like serotonin and dopamine. Deficiencies have been linked to depression and impaired antidepressant response. Vitamin B12 is equally critical for nerve function and red blood cell production, and deficiencies can mimic psychiatric symptoms such as confusion, cognitive decline, and depressive symptoms.

Thyroid function is another crucial piece of the puzzle. The thyroid acts like the body's thermostat, regulating energy, metabolism, and mood. Hypothyroidism can manifest as low energy, slowed thinking, and flat mood, while hyperthyroidism can trigger anxiety, restlessness, and disrupted sleep. Both conditions are sometimes misdiagnosed as psychiatric disorders, which is why comprehensive thyroid testing is essential in mental health evaluations.

It's important to remember that none of these issues exist in isolation. You could be doing all the right things—working on your mindset, applying therapy techniques, practicing mindfulness—and still feel like you're barely staying afloat. In such cases, it's worth asking whether something physical might be making your progress harder than it needs to be. Addressing these deficiencies won't eliminate all challenges, but it will give your mind and body a stronger, more stable foundation. With proper support, energy can return, sleep can deepen, and coping strategies can take root more effectively. This is a critical reminder: Mental health isn't just about what's going on in your thoughts. It's also deeply connected to what's happening in your blood, your cells, and your hormones.

4.8 Key Takeaways: Understanding and Managing the Size of Your Bucket

By now you've taken a closer look at the underlying forces that shape your capacity to handle stress—what I've been referring to as the size of your "mental health bucket." You've explored a range of factors including genetic vulnerabilities, natural temperament, chronic medical conditions, socioeconomic pressures, family dynamics, unresolved trauma, and even biological deficiencies. These are not just abstract theories; they represent the lived realities that either strengthen your ability to cope or quietly shrink your capacity.

If you're beginning to recognize that much of this was set into motion long before you had any say in it, that's exactly the point. One of the most important truths to carry forward from this section is that your mental health capacity is not a reflection of your effort, ambition, or worth. Many of the influences that shape how you experience stress, emotion, and challenge are rooted in aspects of your life you didn't choose—your biology, your upbringing, and your circumstances. So if you've ever felt like you should "just handle it better" or questioned why you struggle when others seem to coast through life effortlessly, this is your invitation to let go of that judgment. It's not weakness. It's wiring.

The goal isn't to erase your past or deny your limitations. The goal is to understand them—and then work with what you've got. The first step is recognizing what's true for you. When certain parts of your story can't be changed—such as your family history, a traumatic experience, or a lifelong medical diagnosis—awareness becomes your most powerful ally. Understanding your personal blueprint allows you to prepare better, recover faster, and respond with greater clarity. Perhaps your nervous system is wired to be more sensitive, or maybe your environment shaped you to be more alert to danger or prone to anxiety. Knowing these truths isn't a life sentence—it's a roadmap.

Recognition is the first, and sometimes the only, step we can take toward certain limitations.

Recognition is the first, and sometimes the only, step we can take toward certain limitations. It can also open the door for planning ahead. You can begin to anticipate what overwhelms you, make adjustments to your environment, and build in safeguards. It also invites more compassion toward yourself. When you find yourself reacting more strongly than expected, you can pause, breathe, and remind yourself that this is part of how you were shaped. That single moment of insight can significantly reduce the internal pressure.

Next, it's time to work with what can be changed. Some aspects of your capacity are surprisingly modifiable, especially when approached with the right tools and support. For example, addressing medical deficiencies such as low Vitamin D or B12, hormonal imbalances, or thyroid dysfunction can dramatically improve your baseline functioning by restoring energy, focus, and mood.

Trauma, while deeply personal and complex, doesn't have to remain a permanent fixture in your narrative. With appropriate support—whether through therapy, trauma-informed care, or body-based practices like mindfulness—you can loosen its emotional grip. The past doesn't vanish, but it becomes less dominant in your daily life.

Even parts of your social environment can shift, if not overnight then gradually. With intention and guidance, you might access new community supports, pursue educational opportunities, or find work that better aligns with your mental health needs. These types of changes can expand your emotional bandwidth and reduce the daily friction that silently fills your bucket. In these ways, your bucket can be strengthened—slowly, intentionally, brick by brick.

Finally, you must learn to adapt where you must. Not every stressor can be eliminated. Not every environment can be controlled. But you can still learn to navigate within your limits. You can make new choices—about your relationships, your boundaries, your routines, and the support systems you lean on. By putting the right structures in place, you can make life more manageable, even when the stressors themselves remain.

This is where your story starts to shift—not by trying to become someone else with a different capacity, but by learning how to live well within the one you have. You're not just learning about stress. You're learning about your capacity for it. You're not just identifying vulnerabilities. You're discovering how to meet them with strategy, support, and strength.

Now you're ready to explore the next layer: the daily factors that either overwhelm your system or help release the pressure. These are the inputs and drains in the Mental Health Bucket Model—what pours in, what flows out, and what tends to linger. Even if your bucket is small, it doesn't have to overflow. And even if your bucket is large, it can still spill over if it's filled too quickly or too often. The key isn't just to understand your structure but to learn how to manage the flow.

So ask yourself: What's currently pouring into your bucket? What do you rely on to release that pressure? And are you holding more than you realize?

In the next chapter, you'll begin examining these inputs—those external demands, pressures, and expectations that accumulate over time. Some are obvious. Others are subtle. However, all of them matter. The clearer you can see what fills your bucket, the more prepared you'll be to protect your balance.

You are building something important here: awareness, clarity, and control. And you're doing it one insight at a time.

The SWOT Exercise: Understanding Your Strengths and Weaknesses

Now that you've examined what shapes the size of your bucket—your innate and environmental capacity for stress—it's time to shift into a more strategic mindset. Awareness is powerful, but awareness paired with structure can transform insight into action. One of the simplest yet most effective frameworks for this next step comes from the world of engineering and organizational strategy: the strengths, weaknesses, opportunities, and threats (SWOT) analysis.[43,44,45]

Originally developed for business and project planning, the SWOT framework helps teams identify internal and external factors that influence performance. It stands for strengths, weaknesses, opportunities, and threats—a four-quadrant map that guides analysis and decision-making. In organizations, it's used to evaluate what's working well, where vulnerabilities lie, what external advantages can be leveraged, and what external risks require mitigation. When applied to your mental health, it becomes a remarkably clarifying exercise in self-understanding.

Here's how it translates on a personal level:

- Strengths represent the aspects of your bucket that naturally enhance resilience or stability. These might include a supportive family, physical health, spiritual grounding, strong emotional insight, or access to care. Think of these as the reinforcements that make your bucket sturdier.
- Weaknesses capture the internal factors that make your system more vulnerable. Maybe you have a history of anxiety, chronic pain, a challenging family dynamic, or trauma. These are the thin spots in your bucket's walls—areas that may need extra attention or reinforcement.
- Opportunities highlight external conditions that could expand your capacity or improve balance. This might include access to therapy, a new community resource, professional mentorship, or upcoming changes that allow for greater rest or flexibility. These are your chances to strengthen or widen the bucket over time.

- Threats identify external stressors or circumstances that could overfill or damage your bucket if left unchecked—such as financial strain, toxic work environments, caregiving burdens, or social isolation. Recognizing them early allows you to build protective barriers before they spill over.

Try this exercise:

Draw a simple square divided into four boxes. Label each one with a SWOT category. Then, looking back over what you've uncovered about your bucket size, begin listing the elements that belong in each quadrant. Which of your traits, circumstances, or patterns serve as strengths? Which ones limit or strain you? What opportunities could you nurture to grow your capacity? And what threats should you monitor or buffer against?

The goal isn't to fix everything at once. It's to see the full system clearly—to visualize your capacity not as a flaw to correct, but as a structure you can understand, maintain, and fortify. This exercise gives you a framework for targeted growth: to build upon what's strong, reinforce what's weak, pursue what's promising, and prepare for what's challenging.

In doing so, you transform your bucket from something that merely reacts to stress into something that evolves with it.

Visit TheBucketModel.com for a free printable download of this exercise and more.

Case Study: When Memory Falters—Uncovering the Hidden Culprit

Dana didn't notice the shift right away. There wasn't one dramatic moment or a clear breaking point. It started quietly, with subtle signs that something was off. She had always been sharp—the kind of leader others relied on in the chaos of tight deadlines and shifting priorities. She was quick with decisions, thorough with details, and known for her ability to juggle a dozen threads of a project in her mind without missing a beat. That had always been Dana's rhythm. Until, suddenly, it wasn't.

Emails began to blur together. She would read them but couldn't recall what they said. In meetings, her mind drifted, and she found herself asking colleagues to repeat things she used to absorb instantly. At first, she chalked it up to stress—a tough quarter, too much on her plate. She believed it would pass. But then she began forgetting even the basics: follow-up calls, important meetings, her niece's birthday dinner. Sticky notes multiplied across her desk. Reminders pinged from her phone. And still, things slipped through the cracks.

The worst part was that people were beginning to notice—her team, her boss. Beneath her calm exterior, panic started to grow. Dana eventually reached out for help. She described the mental fog, the memory lapses, and the creeping anxiety. The initial diagnosis was burnout—executive fatigue. These were classic symptoms of a high performer running on empty. The recommended steps were familiar: improve sleep, reduce screen time, practice mindfulness, lower caffeine, take breaks. She did all of it. Yet things continued to get worse.

Dana started forgetting entire conversations. She would read an email and moments later couldn't remember what it said—or if she had even seen it. The symptoms felt deeper, more frightening. Was this cognitive decline? Early dementia? Her doctor ordered standard labs and began discussing neurological referrals. Dana felt like she was in free fall.

But before diving into expensive neurological testing, her clinician decided to run a full metabolic panel, including basic vitamin levels. It was a small test—but it changed everything. Dana's folic acid levels were significantly low. The cause? A strict ketogenic diet she had started a few months earlier, intended to boost her energy and focus. In significantly cutting out carbohydrates, she had unknowingly eliminated key folate-rich foods such as leafy greens, legumes, and fortified grains.

Folate isn't just a nutrient—it's essential for healthy brain function. Without it, neurotransmitter production falters and cognitive symptoms begin to appear, including attention issues, memory gaps, and mood changes. That's exactly what had been happening to Dana.

With high-dose folic acid supplements and a few dietary adjustments, she slowly began to feel a shift. At first, it was subtle. The fog began to lift. Her mind felt clearer. She no longer needed as many reminders. Her confidence started to return. That familiar sense of mental sharpness—the quality that had once defined her—came back. Three months later, she sat across from her doctor and said, "I'm back! I honestly thought I was losing my mind."

Dana's experience reveals something crucial. Sometimes the issue isn't the faucet pouring too much stress into your bucket—it's the bucket itself, quietly shrinking in the background and limiting your capacity to handle what used to feel routine. Her story is a reminder to pause and look inward when things don't feel right. Not everything is mental. Not everything is about pushing through, trying harder, or assuming you're just burned out.

In Dana's case, the problem wasn't pressure—it was a missing foundation. It was a biological need that, when unmet, compromised her ability to think clearly, regulate emotions, and feel like herself. And it's easy to miss, because on the surface, she was doing everything right. She was managing her stress, getting rest, practicing mindfulness. But without the nutrients her brain required, none of those strategies could fully take root.

It's easy to overlook the physical side of mental health. But when the fog won't lift, when focus keeps slipping, when anxiety starts to feel permanent, it's worth asking: Is my bucket smaller than it used to be? Am I missing something essential? The answer won't always be obvious. But sometimes it's not about more coping—it's about restoration. It's about giving your body and brain what they need to function.

And once you do, clarity returns. Not all at once, but steadily—like sunlight filtering back through clouds that had lingered too long. Dana didn't need a breakthrough. She just needed one missing piece. Sometimes that's all one needs.

Key Takeaway:

Dana's story illustrates that burnout isn't always about too much stress—it can also come from too little support at the biological level. What looked like cognitive overload turned out to be a nutritional deficiency quietly shrinking her capacity to cope. Her case reminds us that the mind and body are inseparable systems; when one falters, the other follows.

The lesson is simple but profound: Not every mental fog is emotional, and not every decline in focus is psychological. Sometimes the bucket isn't overflowing—it's simply smaller than it used to be. Before assuming exhaustion means weakness or poor resilience, it's worth exploring the physical foundations that sustain mental health: sleep, hormones, nutrition, and metabolic balance.

Dana's recovery began not with therapy or time off but with restoration—replenishing what her system lacked. Once her body had what it needed, her mind followed. Burnout recovery isn't always about doing less; sometimes it's about rebuilding from the inside out.

5

The Inputs (Faucets)

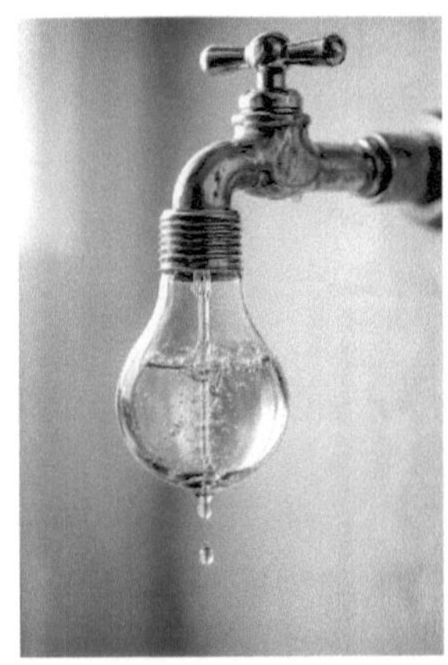

UP TO THIS point, you've explored what determines the size of your bucket—your unique ability to absorb stress before it starts to spill over. Now it's time to shift focus. Because even the strongest, most resilient bucket can only hold so much. What truly tests its limits is what flows into it: the daily pressures, challenges, and emotional demands that accumulate over time. These stressors are your faucets.

Understanding your faucets is just as important as knowing your capacity. A small bucket might stay steady if the flow is light. But even a large one can overflow if too many faucets are gushing at once. This is where the concepts of volume and frequency become especially helpful. Volume reflects how much stress each faucet releases. Is it just a drip, or does it feel like a pressure washer turned on high? A minor inconvenience might add a few drops, while a serious financial setback might unleash a flood. Frequency, on the other hand, speaks to how often the faucet turns on. Is it a once-a-month issue that catches you off guard, or is it something that runs in the background every single day?

Together, volume and frequency shape how full your bucket becomes—not just in a moment but over time. A single high-volume event might take a while to recover from, while a dozen low-volume, high-frequency stressors can quietly wear you down without warning. The key is awareness. You don't need to shut off every faucet—but once you see them clearly, you can begin to control the flow. In the next section, you'll begin identifying your own faucets—the ones you've accepted as normal, the ones you didn't realize were still on, and the ones you might finally be ready to adjust.

You don't need to shut off every faucet—but once you see them clearly, you can begin to control the flow.

5.1 Why Volume and Frequency Matter

To understand how stress builds up over time, imagine two different types of faucets. One faucet releases a heavy stream of water, but it only turns on occasionally—perhaps during a crisis or a major life event. This is a high-volume, low-frequency faucet. When it flows, it hits hard and fast. The second faucet, in contrast, emits a slow, quiet trickle of water, but it runs every single day. At first it may seem barely noticeable, but over time, it can fill the bucket just as much. This is a low-volume, high-frequency source of stress.

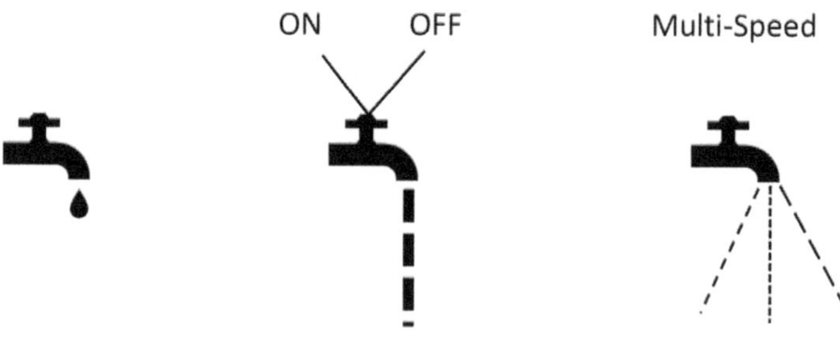

Both types of stress can overwhelm your system, but they do so in very different ways. The high-volume stress might cause an acute spike that demands immediate attention, whereas the low-volume, daily stressors often go unnoticed until your reserves are drained and signs of burnout appear unexpectedly. The key to managing either type is to recognize them for what they are and understand how much each one contributes to your overall load.

To make this practical, consider mapping out your personal stress landscape. Begin by listing all the current stressors in your life. Be honest and thorough—no matter how large or small a stressor may seem, if it takes up space in your mental or emotional life, it matters. These stressors might include relationship struggles; financial pressures; health issues; major life changes; experiences of loss, grief, or uncertainty; the relentless pull of responsibilities or social comparison; and even environmental factors like social media, the news, or background noise.

Once you have your list, examine each stressor through two key lenses: how often it appears (its frequency) and how intense it feels when it does (its volume). With those factors in mind, you can begin placing each stressor into a simple matrix that helps you visualize their cumulative effect, with the below diagram highlighting some examples:

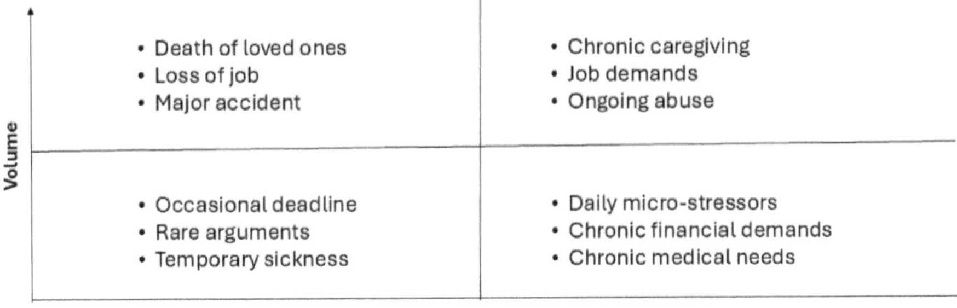

This visual mapping offers more than insight—it provides clarity. It helps you identify which stressors pour the most into your bucket, highlighting where the greatest pressure lies and pointing to areas where small or large changes might offer the most relief. Depending on context and control, high-frequency, high-volume stressors demand your highest priority.

It's also essential to remember that comparing stress buckets with others is rarely helpful. There's no universal scale that dictates how much a particular stressor "should" affect someone. What feels manageable to one person might be completely overwhelming to another, depending on their history, temperament, and current state of well-being. For instance, two individuals might both experience health issues—one dealing with chronic low-grade pain, and the other facing severe but sporadic flare-ups. Both experiences are valid, and both take up emotional space in different ways.

So when you look at your own stress matrix, try to release any urge to compare your struggles with someone else's. There's no "right" way to feel—only your reality as it stands. The goal of this exercise is not to be perfect but to become more aware of your unique stress landscape.

Keep in mind that stressors are not fixed. They evolve with time. Some stress faucets will naturally turn off or slow to a drip. Others may surge open without warning. Relationships change. Jobs begin or end. Health conditions improve or worsen. Even your response to a familiar stressor might shift depending on your age, emotional state, or current life season.

That's why this matrix should not be treated as a one-time reflection. It is a living tool—something to revisit whenever your life feels out of balance. As your circumstances change, so does the way your bucket fills. By regularly checking in with this framework, you can better anticipate what overwhelms you, protect your energy, and restore balance before burnout takes root.

5.2 The Nervous System: Your Body's Response to Stressful Inputs

By now you've seen how inputs—or stressors—begin to fill your mental health bucket. But what exactly is happening inside your body when those stress faucets turn on? Every time you perceive a threat—whether it's a missed deadline, a tense conversation, or simply another doomscroll through the news—your body reacts using a built-in system designed to protect you: the autonomic nervous system.[1,2,3]

This system functions like the controls of a car, with two primary branches. The sympathetic nervous system acts as your internal gas pedal, responsible for the "fight-or-flight" response. The parasympathetic nervous system, on the other hand, serves as the brake pedal, responsible for "rest and digest." Both are essential, and maintaining balance between them is key to resilience. The challenge lies in knowing when to accelerate and when to slow down.

When your brain senses stress or danger—whether physical or psychological—it presses the gas. The sympathetic nervous system ramps up the body to meet the challenge. Heart rate and blood pressure rise, delivering more blood to your muscles. Breathing becomes quicker and shallower to increase oxygen intake. Digestion slows, since it's deprioritized during perceived danger. Cortisol and adrenaline surge, keeping you alert and focused. Your muscles tense in preparation to fight-or-flight, and immune function drops as the body diverts energy from long-term repair to immediate survival.

This sympathetic response is helpful when it's short-lived and targeted. But in today's world, where chronic stress is the norm, it often stays switched on. Continuous activation—driven by overwork, lack of sleep, nonstop notifications, and information overload—leads to physical and emotional exhaustion. Instead of feeling alert and focused, you begin to feel foggy, drained, and irritable. Your body and brain simply can't sustain that pace indefinitely.

That's where the parasympathetic system comes in. This "brake" helps your body rest, recover, and reset. It supports digestion, tissue repair, deep sleep, and a general sense of calm. In a well-regulated nervous system, you naturally shift between sympathetic and parasympathetic modes. You accelerate when needed and then slow down to recover. But when stress inputs keep piling up and there's no space to ease off the gas, you get stuck in high gear. And that's when things start to break down.

The challenge we face today is that our nervous systems haven't evolved as quickly as our environment. They still respond to everyday inputs—emails, missed calls, social media alerts—as if they are life-threatening. Unlike the saber-toothed tigers of the past, these modern stressors don't resolve quickly. They repeat, persist, and even follow us in our pockets. This constant low-grade activation keeps your body on alert, your foot on the gas, and your system overheating. It's one of the core reasons burnout feels not just emotional but physical.

Understanding how your nervous system responds to stress is more than just interesting—it's vital. As we move forward and explore more about the different types of stress inputs (including job misalignment, news, and social media), you'll begin to see that stress affects more than just your mood. It initiates biological reactions that shape your energy, focus, sleep, digestion, immunity, and overall well-being.

The good news is that once you learn to recognize what's pressing on your gas pedal—and how to intentionally engage your brakes—you'll begin to regain control. You can begin to regulate your stress responses rather than be ruled by them. And that's exactly where we're headed next.

5.3 Job Misalignment: When Work Becomes a Faucet with Multiple Settings

Work is one of the most persistent sources of stress in many people's lives. While some stressors—like family conflict, financial pressure, or health concerns—are easy to identify, work often becomes the faucet that runs the most. It's not just because of long hours or demanding expectations. Work touches nearly every area of life: time, energy, identity, purpose. When your work aligns with your strengths and values, it can energize and fulfill you. But when there's a mismatch—when it drains you without giving anything back—it can run endlessly in the background, steadily filling your mental health bucket.

The good news is that once you learn to recognize what's pressing on your gas pedal—and how to intentionally engage your brakes—you'll begin to regain control.

Burnout isn't always about doing too much. Often it's about doing too much of what doesn't fit. Christina Maslach's research reframes burnout not as a personal failure but as a mismatch between the individual and their job.[4] Her framework identifies six key domains of workplace misalignment that create ideal conditions for burnout. You can think of your job faucet as having six spray settings—each one representing a different part of your work experience. Each setting can either support you or wear you down.

The first setting is *workload*, or the high-pressure jet. This one is hard to miss. When demands pile up without pause—too many meetings, constant deadlines, unrealistic expectations—it leaves you feeling like you can never catch up. Even when the workday ends, your mind stays active, rehearsing to-do lists or worrying about unfinished tasks. It's not just about being busy—it's about the feeling that rest is always out of reach.

The second setting is *control*, or the unpredictable spray. It's not the amount of work, but the lack of autonomy that causes strain. When you don't feel like you have a say in your schedule, decisions, or approach, it creates chronic tension. Flexibility turns into fatigue. Control isn't about total authority—it's about having enough agency to feel steady. Without that, even quiet moments can leave you feeling on edge.

The third domain is *reward*, the drip that shouldn't matter—but does. You give your best, show up consistently, and contribute meaningfully, but receive little recognition. The reward faucet isn't just about salary—it's about feeling seen, appreciated, and valued. When that's absent, it gradually chips away at motivation. It may not be dramatic, but over time, it drains your energy and sense of worth.

The fourth is *community*, the uneven spray. This setting reflects your relationships at work. If you're surrounded by tension, conflict, exclusion, or coldness, it becomes harder to feel grounded. You don't need deep friendships with coworkers, but you do need to feel like you belong. Disconnection at work doesn't always feel like sadness—it can show up as irritability, disengagement, or the desire to emotionally shut down.

The fifth domain is *fairness*, or the tilted stream. This shows up when others are praised for the same work you do, when decisions feel inconsistent or biased, or when rules change depending on who's asking. Lack of fairness erodes trust. Without trust, psychological safety disappears. And without safety, your nervous system stays on high alert. Unpredictability is its own form of stress.

The sixth and final setting is *values*, the off-center stream. This misalignment is often more subtle, but deeply draining. When your work doesn't reflect what matters to you—when it feels disconnected from your purpose—it creates internal friction. You may begin to feel out of place or disconnected from yourself. That kind of misalignment leads to a type of fatigue that rest alone can't fix.

Domain	Faucet Analogy	Description	Impact on Well-Being
Workload	High-pressure jet	Constant demands, excessive meetings, deadlines, and expectations	Creates mental overload and the sense that rest is never achievable
Control	Unpredictable spray	Lack of autonomy in decisions, schedules, or methods	Leads to chronic tension, anxiety, and reduced sense of stability
Reward	The unnoticed drip	Limited recognition or appreciation despite effort and consistency	Gradual erosion of motivation and self-worth
Community	Uneven spray	Conflict, exclusion, or emotional coldness in workplace relationships	Results in disengagement, irritability, and emotional withdrawal
Fairness	Tilted stream	Biased decision-making, inconsistent rules, or lack of equity in recognition or treatment	Undermines trust and psychological safety, keeping the nervous system on alert
Values	Off-center stream	Mismatch between personal values and the nature or purpose of one's work	Generates internal conflict and existential fatigue that rest alone cannot repair

One faulty spray setting might not overwhelm your system. But when several of these misalignments pile up—when workload is unmanageable, control is lacking, and your values feel compromised—it creates a relentless flow that steadily fills your bucket. This is why burnout often creeps in rather than crashes down. It builds gradually, unnoticed, until everything feels too heavy.

You don't have to solve every problem at once. But understanding these six domains offers clarity and language for what you're experiencing. It's the first step toward change.

Before moving on, take a moment to reflect: Is your job faucet running too fast? Which of these six settings feels most misaligned? What's one small adjustment you could make to ease the pressure? It may not mean switching jobs altogether. Sometimes the answer is a subtle shift in how you approach your work, where you direct your energy, or how you advocate for support. Even a small recalibration can make a meaningful difference.

Up next, you'll examine another modern faucet—one that never seems to turn off: the digital world. The constant influx of news, notifications, and social media may be adding more stress to your bucket than you realize.

5.4 News: A High-Frequency, Often High-Volume Faucet

The digital world doesn't pause—and neither does the news. What was once a contained part of the day, such as a morning paper or an evening broadcast, has transformed into a nonstop stream of information. Breaking headlines, live updates, and constant notifications buzz from your pocket throughout the day. While the intention behind staying informed might feel responsible, the outcome is often overstimulation, emotional exhaustion, and a heaviness that seems to appear without an obvious cause.

In the context of the Mental Health Bucket Model, news consumption represents a unique kind of faucet. It's quiet, frequent, and often more intense than anticipated. Unlike situational stressors—like a missed deadline or a tense conversation—the news doesn't wait for a major event to turn on. It's always present, always dripping, and often focused on what's going wrong in the world.

The frequency of news exposure is relentless. You might scroll headlines while brushing your teeth, check breaking news at a red light, or read about natural disasters just before bed. This constant exposure to global stress is a form of high-frequency stress. It blurs the boundary between your personal world and the wider one, training your brain to stay hypervigilant. You may even find yourself anticipating bad news before unlocking your phone.

It's not just how often you consume the news—it's the volume and emotional impact of the stories themselves.[5] Topics like mass shootings, political division, injustice, and environmental catastrophe carry significant emotional weight. Even when these stories don't affect you directly, they can still leave a mark through a process called *vicarious trauma*—stress absorbed through empathy.[6,7] Each heartbreaking report quietly adds to your already full mental load.

Your brain was never meant to process this much distress at once. One moment it's inflation, the next it's war, then a scandal, a virus, or a new climate warning. The onslaught leaves no time for reflection or emotional processing, just a conveyor belt of anxiety-provoking information. The result is mental confusion, emotional fragmentation, and a deepening sense of helplessness—all of which drain energy and increase stress.[8]

This constant barrage of emotionally charged content keeps your nervous system on high alert. News stories are designed to provoke—anger, fear, outrage—because those emotions drive engagement.[9] But every emotional reaction also triggers a physiological one: Adrenaline surges, cortisol rises, and muscles tense. When there's no resolution or moment of pause, your body never truly powers down. The long-term effect? Fatigue, irritability, sleeplessness, and even physical discomfort.

Burnout doesn't always stem from loud, dramatic events. It often grows from chronic, low-grade pressure—and the news fits that description perfectly. Over time, you might find yourself withdrawing from things you once enjoyed, feeling numb or disconnected from others, or compulsively consuming more news in the hope of understanding what's going on—even as you feel worse after doing so. The problems begin to feel too big, and your capacity to care starts to collapse under the weight.

Burnout doesn't always stem from loud, dramatic events. It often grows from chronic, low-grade pressure—and the news fits that description perfectly.

The issue isn't being informed—it's absorbing news without processing it. Most headlines are designed to hook your attention and provoke emotion, not to empower you. They rarely offer actionable steps or closure. If you read something, can't do anything about it, but carry the emotional burden anyway, you've added to your stress without any release.

You don't have to unplug completely, but you do need boundaries.[10] Set a specific window of time during the day to catch up on the news—ideally not right when you wake up or before bed. Choose a few reputable sources that prioritize clarity over sensationalism. Turn off news alerts, which hijack your nervous system with every ping. Before diving into a story, ask yourself, *Can I act on this?* If not, it might be healthier to let it go. Balance news consumption with grounding activities like walking, reading, journaling, or spending time with people. And regularly check in with your body—notice how certain stories affect your tension, breath, or energy. Use that awareness to protect your peace.

Remember, the news doesn't just inform—it impacts. In a world that never stops talking, silence is still an option. You're not required to carry the weight of the world. You're allowed to step back, even momentarily, and give your nervous system the break it deserves. Your mind and body will thank you.

5.5 Social Media: The Double-Edged Faucet

Social media doesn't announce itself—it quietly seeps into your daily life. Whether it's Instagram, TikTok, Facebook, LinkedIn, or the infinite scroll of X (formerly Twitter), it's always present. It shows up in the in-between moments, during periods of rest, and even during the night, through the glow of your screen. While it appears to offer connection, distraction, amusement, or even comfort, it also serves as a faucet that rarely turns off. This faucet steadily drips—or sometimes gushes—into your mental health bucket, often without you realizing how much it adds until you're overwhelmed.

Social media doesn't require a specific trigger to affect you. It only asks for a glance, a swipe, or a scroll. These seemingly small moments, repeated dozens or hundreds of times a day, keep your mind in a constant state of stimulation. Unlike other stressors that demand a clear cause, social media's impact is sustained by habit. It invades the time once reserved for silence—during meals, breaks, and downtime. Even if you think you're "just checking," your brain is constantly processing new information, switching tasks, reacting to comparisons, and absorbing headlines. The space that could have supported rest or reflection instead becomes cluttered with noise.

Emotionally, social media can be chaotic.[11] One post may make you laugh, the next may spark envy, and another may provoke outrage or grief. Social media's emotional whiplash overwhelms your nervous system, which was never designed to switch so rapidly between such intense reactions. Over time, this leads to chronic low-grade tension. You may feel restless, wired, and disconnected from your own baseline—your inner calm.

A major contributor to this emotional toll is the constant invitation to compare yourself with others. Social media showcases curated glimpses of people's lives—career achievements, beautiful relationships, well-decorated homes—which, though filtered and edited, still influence how you see yourself.[12] You may begin to feel inadequate or left behind, not because your life is lacking but because your perspective has been distorted by unrealistic portrayals. The more you seek validation or connection through social media, the more fragile your self-worth becomes. It starts to depend on engagement—likes, comments, shares—turning identity into a performance rather than a reflection of your reality.

Although social media promises a break from the day, it rarely delivers genuine restoration. The infinite scroll offers no natural stopping point. What begins as a few minutes quickly becomes an hour, replacing true rest with mental clutter. Focus weakens, attention fragments, and your recovery time vanishes. The energy you could have used to decompress is instead spent reacting to content that leaves you more exhausted than before.

This persistent stimulation contributes to burnout. Social media's negative impact may not always feel obvious or dramatic. Instead, it manifests subtly—through emotional fatigue, difficulty concentrating, a lack of presence in relationships, and a compulsive urge to check your device. These are quiet signs, but they add up. Burnout doesn't require one major crisis—it can arise from constant, low-level pressure over time.

You don't need to abandon social media entirely, but setting boundaries can help you regain control.[13] Consider limiting your social media use to specific times of day, especially avoiding it in the morning and before bed. Turn off notifications to protect your nervous system from unnecessary alerts. Curate your feed—follow accounts that uplift you and unfollow those that drain your energy. Before scrolling, ask yourself whether you're seeking connection or information, or simply avoiding discomfort. Replace screen time with more restorative habits, such as walking, journaling, or having a real conversation. Even taking short breaks from social media, such as a day or weekend off, can reset your nervous system and improve your clarity.

Ultimately, social media is not inherently harmful, but it's not neutral either. It is a tool—and like any tool, its impact depends on how it's used. You don't need to reject it altogether, but you should be intentional about when and how it enters your life. If your mental health bucket feels unusually full, look to your screen time. Consider how often your attention is hijacked and how little space is left for your own thoughts. You deserve a mind that isn't constantly reacting, a life free from constant comparison, and a rhythm that includes genuine rest. Adjusting this faucet—one mindful choice at a time—is a good place to start.

5.6 Inputs: Takeaways and Management Strategies

Your bucket can only hold so much. To protect your mental and emotional space, it's important to be honest about what's flowing in and recognize where you still have control. Some stressors are within reach—these are the ones you can influence, prioritize, adjust, or even eliminate. Others exist outside your control, regardless of how much effort or worry you invest. Learning to distinguish between the two is where true resilience begins.

Managing the things that pour into your bucket requires a three-part approach. First, identify them, put names to them, and characterize them while understanding their respective volume and frequency into your life. This recognition is the most powerful first step toward addressing them, as often noted in the engineering adage: "A problem well-defined is half solved."[14]

Second, prioritize and reduce what you can. This means turning down—or turning off—the stressors within your sphere of influence. It might look like setting firmer boundaries at work, limiting social media exposure, stepping away from commitments that no longer serve you, or having a long-overdue conversation that clears the air. Each of these actions lightens your load, even in small ways. The goal isn't to eliminate all stress but to stop treating fixable problems as if they're permanent fixtures in your life.

Third, learn how to work with what cannot be changed. Certain stressors such as illness, loss, or major life transitions won't disappear no matter how much you wish they would. These are the *uncontrollables*. But even in the face of such challenges, you are not helpless. You can shift how you respond to them.

This is where radical acceptance becomes a valuable tool. Radical acceptance means being at peace with realities we cannot change. It doesn't mean giving up or pretending everything is fine. Instead, it means acknowledging reality as it is, without wasting energy fighting what cannot be undone. That acceptance doesn't solve the problem, but it prevents you from depleting yourself through resistance. And the energy you save? You'll need it elsewhere—for healing, for coping, and for simply making it through the day.

Radical acceptance means being at peace with realities we cannot change.

The more often you check in with your internal stress landscape by asking yourself, *Is this something I can control?*, the more grounded and empowered you become. With clarity, your reactions become more measured, and your decisions feel more intentional.

Here are a few truths to carry with you: Not all stressors affect you the same way. Some hit like floods, while others are slow leaks. What matters most is how much they fill you over time. Awareness creates opportunity—identifying a controllable stressor is the first step in reclaiming your energy. Acceptance is not a sign of weakness; it is a powerful way to protect your emotional reserves. This is a skill you can build through mindfulness, self-compassion, and reframing your perspective. Over time, you'll learn to carry the burdens you cannot drop, and release the ones you no longer need to hold.

Reflection offers a chance to reset. Return to your stress map regularly. What once seemed immovable may now be open to change, and what once felt manageable may now require new boundaries.

Your next step is to explore the other side of the equation: the drains—the intentional ways to relieve pressure, restore balance, and give your bucket the relief it needs.

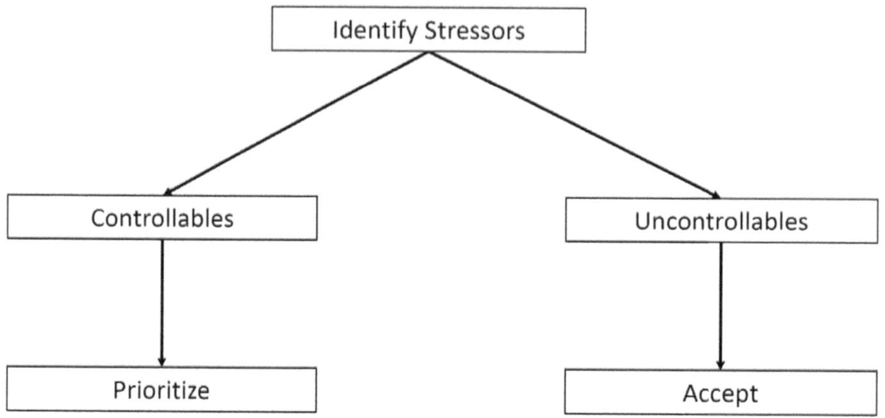

Exercise: Mapping Your Inputs

Before you move on to the next chapter, take a moment to pause and map what's currently pouring into your bucket. Awareness is the starting point for control. This exercise isn't about judging your stressors or labeling them as good or bad—it's about seeing them clearly, as they are. Once they're visible, you can begin to understand their pattern, their weight, and their rhythm.

Start by listing the major inputs in your life—the sources that steadily or suddenly fill your bucket. Some are obvious: work demands, family responsibilities, finances, deadlines, or health concerns. Others are quieter: guilt, perfectionism, self-doubt, or the pressure to meet invisible expectations. Write them down as they come to mind.

Next, consider two dimensions for each input: **volume** and **frequency**.

- *Volume* describes how strongly this stressor affects you when it's active. Some hit like a surge of water from a fire hose; others are light but constant drips.
- *Frequency* refers to how often this faucet runs. Is it always on? Does it appear a few times a week, or only during specific seasons or events?

Now take a closer look. Which of these inputs are within your control? Which can be adjusted, limited, or eliminated with time and intention? And which are beyond your reach—those that require acceptance rather than resistance? The purpose of this reflection is not to fix everything today but to separate what's changeable from what simply needs to be met with grace.

If it helps, draw a simple table with three columns: one for your stress inputs, one for their volume and frequency, and one for whether they are controllable or not. Seeing it on paper often brings clarity. You might notice that a few small but constant drips add up to more pressure than a single major event, or that certain stressors run on autopilot because you've never thought to turn them down.

When you're done, take a step back and review your list. Which inputs deserve attention right now? Which can wait? And which can be released from the illusion of control? That awareness alone can shift your balance more than any drastic change.

You'll return to this map often. Over time, some faucets will quiet down, and others may open unexpectedly. The goal isn't to keep them all off—it's to manage the flow with intention, so your bucket fills more slowly, drains more effectively, and remains steady when life gets loud.

Visit TheBucketModel.com for a free printable download of this exercise and more.

Case Study: When the Commute Becomes the Crisis

A few years into his professional career, Adam appeared to be thriving. As a young, high-achieving worker, he had recently completed his training and secured a position that allowed him to work independently at a satellite location several hours from the main office. Although the long commute wasn't ideal, it initially felt worthwhile. Adam took pride in his work, earned recognition from clients, and was regarded as dependable and driven by his supervisors. The long drives gave him time to think. Life was full, but it felt manageable.

Over time, however, that rhythm began to unravel. Adam's mother, who had been living independently, started showing signs of cognitive decline. What began as minor forgetfulness escalated into wandering, confusion, and unsafe behavior. After months of trial and error—including a taxing period when he attempted to move his mother into his home—Adam made the painful decision to place his mother in a memory care facility. Though it was the safest option, it left him with a persistent emotional weight filled with guilt, grief, and self-doubt.

Soon after, Adam's physical health began to deteriorate. He developed a blood clot and was placed on anticoagulation therapy. Later, he experienced a heart arrhythmia that required surgical intervention. His body was sending unmistakable signals of distress. Aware that the daily commute was further draining his energy and mental bandwidth, Adam formally requested a transfer to a closer site within the same organization. Although the request was approved, the change never materialized.

Days turned into months, and those months stretched into over a year and a half. During that time, things continued to decline. Adam began experiencing panic attacks, his sleep quality plummeted, and his ability to focus diminished. One day, a client threatened him during a routine appointment—an incident that once might have rolled off his back but now triggered a spiral of anxiety. He found it increasingly difficult to separate his internal turmoil from the pressures of his job.

Eventually, Adam sought professional help. In therapy, he began to connect the dots: unresolved grief, chronic health issues, and ongoing workplace misalignment were silently amplifying the stress pouring into his mental health bucket. He started a temporary course of medication to stabilize his symptoms and leaned into therapeutic tools that helped him differentiate between what he could control and what he could not.

One unexpected insight emerged as he reflected on his daily habits: His digital routines were quietly making things worse. In moments of stress or fatigue, Adam would scroll through social media or check news feeds to stay connected or unwind. But rather than providing relief, these habits acted like an unchecked faucet—introducing a constant stream of bad news, polarizing debates, and filtered snapshots of other people's lives. These inputs only deepened his unease and added to his emotional overload.

In response, Adam took a bold step and unplugged. He deleted social media apps from his phone and set strict boundaries around his news intake. Instead, he introduced calming and meaningful content into his routine, such as audiobooks, spiritual talks, and nature sounds during his commute. The result was immediate and noticeable. His nervous system began to settle, his thoughts became less reactive, and his sleep improved.

This digital detox didn't erase his problems, but it created the mental space he needed to address them with greater clarity. One powerful realization emerged: Adam had been waiting too long for change without asserting his needs. With renewed resolve, he approached his employer again—this time with a firm boundary: Either the transfer would happen promptly, or he would begin exploring other job opportunities. Within weeks, the long-delayed relocation was finally implemented.

The shift in his circumstances brought an immediate sense of relief. Working closer to home allowed Adam to reclaim hours of his day. He used that time to restructure his evenings, prioritize sleep, and reintroduce a consistent exercise routine. The panic attacks stopped. His physical health stabilized. In therapy, he learned how to sit with the discomfort of his mother's illness without being overwhelmed by it. He used cognitive behavioral techniques to challenge and reframe his guilt into healthier, more compassionate thoughts. He also reconnected with his spiritual practices, which brought him a deeper sense of peace and meaning.

Adam's transformation didn't stem from eliminating all sources of stress. His job still carried its demands, and his mother's condition continued to weigh on him. But by addressing the most mismatched faucet—his long commute—and reducing the invisible stressors caused by media consumption, he was able to shift the overall flow of stress into his system. These external changes, combined with deliberate internal work, allowed him to reopen the "drains" in his mental health bucket and begin to recover.

Over time, Adam was able to taper off medication. His focus returned. He resumed pursuing professional certifications he had once set aside. Today he is not just functioning—he is thriving. He speaks about his experiences with humility and insight and often mentors colleagues who are facing similar challenges. For the first time in a long while, he is planning his future not from a place of burnout, but from a place of vision and intention.

Key Takeaway:

Adam's story is a powerful reminder that burnout doesn't always come from dramatic overload. Sometimes it arises from slow, persistent misalignment between your needs and your environment. In his case, the issue wasn't a toxic job or a harmful employer—it was a prolonged logistical and emotional strain that became unsustainable. His healing began the moment he stopped waiting passively for things to change and started reclaiming agency over his circumstances.

His journey also highlights how often invisible inputs, like digital media, contribute to emotional exhaustion. Information overload may not feel like stress in the moment, but it erodes the nervous system over time. By removing that stream, Adam made space for his thoughts and emotions to settle.

The path to recovery isn't always about quitting. Sometimes it's about renegotiating terms, setting digital boundaries, and recognizing when it's time to stop asking for change and start requiring it. That's when true healing begins.

6

The Drains

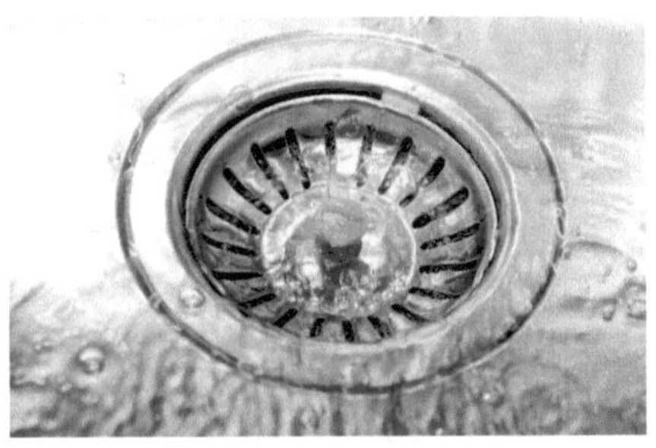

YOU'VE ALREADY SEEN how life's demands can pour into your bucket—through nonstop inputs, stressors, expectations, and emotions that accumulate over time, either as a slow drip or in heavy streams. The more that flows in, the heavier everything begins to feel. But focusing only on what pours in tells only part of the story. What many overlook are the drains.

Your drains are what provide relief. They create space in your system. They don't erase the stress entirely, but they give you the ability to process it, release it, and recover. Without effective drains, your bucket has no off-switch. No matter how strong or resilient you are, or how large your capacity may seem, your bucket will eventually overflow if nothing is allowed to flow out—and that's when burnout takes hold. Understanding your drains isn't just helpful—it's essential.

Drains are the quiet supports you intentionally build into your life.

Drains are the quiet supports you intentionally build into your life. They include the practices, habits, and rhythms that help your nervous system feel safe and grounded again. Drains are how you reset after a long day, how you recover after emotional tension, and how you restore the energy that stress depletes. These aren't luxuries; they are your foundation. Drains help you recover from both emotional and physical stress, clear out the mental fog that accumulates from constant stimulation, reconnect with your body and your thoughts, and rebuild your capacity to cope—so that the next wave of stress doesn't knock you over. The good news is that, unlike most inputs, you have more control over your drains. You may not always choose what flows into your life, but you can choose how well your drains function.

In the chapters ahead, you'll take a closer look at seven powerful, research-backed drains that directly support your mental and emotional well-being.[1,2,3,4] First is sleep—not just the number of hours you spend in bed, but the quality and depth of rest that allows your brain to reset and your body to heal. Without true rest, every stressor feels more intense.

Next is diet. What you feed your body becomes the fuel—or friction—that your mind has to work with. Nutrition affects not only energy levels, but also mood, inflammation, focus, and emotional stability. Then there's exercise. Movement doesn't just affect your physical health, it alters your brain chemistry. Physical activity helps move stress through and out of your system. Even a short walk can significantly turn down the internal noise.

You'll also explore substances. Certain substances can either support your drains or quietly clog them. This section isn't about judgment—it's about gaining awareness and making informed choices that support your overall balance. Mindfulness will be another focus—the intentional practice of bringing your attention back to the present moment. Mindfulness can calm your nervous system, interrupt cycles of anxious thinking, and create inner space even when your external circumstances remain unchanged.

The next topic is habit formation. Sustainable change doesn't rely on willpower alone. It comes from designing routines that support your recovery without requiring constant motivation. Tiny, consistent shifts—done daily—can establish powerful drains over time. Finally, you'll explore social connection. Humans aren't built to carry everything alone. Genuine connection—feeling seen, supported, and safe with others—acts as a shared drain. It helps lighten the load and distributes emotional weight across safe relationships.

These areas are not about striving for perfection. They're about creating enough flow and release to keep your system in balance. A healthy drain doesn't mean that stress disappears altogether—it simply means you're no longer forced to carry it all internally. This next part of your journey is about making space. Not by avoiding life, but by learning how to support your bucket and give it a chance to breathe—one small, intentional drain at a time.

6.1 The Nervous System: Activating Your Body's Natural Drainage System

By now you've seen how stress enters your mental and emotional system—from work demands and relationship tensions to the steady influx of news and the constant presence of your phone. You've also begun to explore the concept of drains—those vital outlets that allow you to release built-up stress. But behind every habit that opens your drains, whether it's rest, movement, or stillness, there is something deeper at work. At the core of this process lies a powerful biological system: the parasympathetic nervous system. This system plays one of the most essential roles in helping your body reset, recover, and heal.[5,6] If the stress response functions like a gas pedal, this system is the brake.

The parasympathetic nervous system is sometimes referred to as the "rest and digest" system. While that nickname may sound casual, it's actually a blueprint for how your body recovers. When this system becomes active, your body begins to send a very different message than it does when you are under stress. That message is simple: You're safe now. You can relax. Once your body receives that signal, it begins the process of repair. Your heart rate slows down and blood pressure drops, leaving you feeling more grounded. Your breathing deepens, allowing more oxygen to enter your system and calming both body and mind. Digestion resumes, as blood flow returns to the gut and allows your internal systems to function properly. Your muscles begin to release tension, your jaw unclenches, your shoulders drop, and your chest opens. Stress hormones like cortisol decrease, while brain chemistry shifts toward calm and connection. Even your immune system benefits—inflammation reduces, and your body moves from defense mode to a state of readiness and restoration. In short, your entire system says: Now is the time to heal.

The parasympathetic nervous system is sometimes referred to as the "rest and digest" system.

Despite the power of the parasympathetic system, it doesn't activate on its own—especially if you're living in a state of constant low-grade stress. You may tell yourself to relax, but if your body is still braced and your mind is still racing, very little actually shifts. This is why real relaxation—true, restorative recovery—is different from simply zoning out in front of a screen. It requires intentional effort. It may even require repetition and practice. This is where daily habits come into play. Things like restful sleep, nourishing food, gentle movement, and stillness are not just good ideas—they are biological signals. Each time you engage in one of these habits, you're teaching your nervous system what safety feels like. And once your body knows it's safe, it knows how to let go.

Managing stress isn't about eliminating life's challenges. Rather, it's about strengthening your system's ability to recover. Each time you slow your breath, move your body, nourish it well, or allow yourself to rest, you send a powerful internal message: *You're not in danger. You don't need to brace yourself constantly. You're allowed to release.* This message doesn't just provide momentary relief. Over time, it reshapes your internal baseline. It builds resilience and expands your capacity to carry life's inevitable stressors without breaking.

Without functioning drains, even minor stressors can accumulate. Your body never gets the message to reset. Over time, this leads to restless sleep, low mood, poor focus, and physical exhaustion—even if you're technically "resting." You may find yourself feeling wired but tired, your body still on high alert even when you're safe at home. That's why this next part of your journey is more than a list of wellness tips—it's a deliberate effort to reclaim your body's internal balance. Your nervous system isn't broken. It isn't the enemy. It has simply been overstimulated for too long.

In the next chapters, you'll begin exploring the most powerful and proven drains that help regulate your nervous system and restore balance. You'll start with sleep—because when sleep returns, many other areas of health and emotional stability begin to align. From there, you'll continue building a toolkit of habits that support your mind and body in letting go, healing, and thriving.

6.2 Sleep

Sleep is the most foundational drain in your mental health system. It's not just about rest—it's about repair. When your mood, focus, or energy feel off, the problem often starts with sleep. Your body sees sleep as a restoration window, a time to clear out the mental and physical mess left behind by your day. If you miss that window or cut it short, it's like skipping the cleanup after a storm. The debris builds, the clutter compounds, and slowly your bucket begins to fill.

Sleep can simply be described as your maintenance mode.[7,8,9] Even though the lights are off, essential work is happening behind the scenes. Your brain detoxes as the lymphatic system kicks in, essentially rinsing your mind and clearing out waste built up from stress, stimulation, and decision-making. Your memory sharpens as sleep stabilizes what you've learned, helping you retain information and make better decisions. Your immune system recharges as inflammation decreases, making your body more resilient to illness and stress. Your emotions also settle—cortisol levels drop, mood-regulating chemicals reset, and you wake up feeling steadier and calmer. Without enough sleep, this entire system breaks down.[10] You might feel edgy, scattered, or overly reactive. Even a small sleep deficit can amplify anxiety, cloud your thinking, and make minor setbacks feel overwhelming.

Sleep can simply be described as your maintenance mode.

The issue is that sleep is often the first thing sacrificed. Late-night scrolling, unfinished tasks, and endless distractions eat away at the one thing your body needs most to stay balanced. And when sleep suffers, everything else begins to suffer too.

For most adults, the sweet spot for sleep is between seven and nine hours per night. But it's not just about the number—it's about rhythm, quality, and consistency. Building a healthy sleep routine means training your body to expect rest and creating the right conditions to allow that rest to happen. One way to do this is by setting a consistent sleep window. Pick a wake-up time and count backward about eight hours to find your ideal bedtime. Stick to this schedule as much as possible, even on weekends. Your body thrives on rhythm, and regularity strengthens your internal clock.

An hour before bed, begin winding down.[11] This is your soft landing, signaling to your nervous system that it's safe to slow down. Put away screens, since blue light and constant input can trick your brain into staying alert. Replace scrolling with a book, journal, or calming audio. Cool your room, as sleep often comes easier in a slightly cooler environment. You can adjust the thermostat, use a fan, or crack a window. Ease your body with progressive muscle relaxation—tensing and releasing muscle groups from head to toe—or take a warm bath or shower. As your core temperature drops afterward, you'll naturally feel sleepier. Calming sounds such as nature recordings, white noise, or spiritual melodies can further soothe your mind and anchor your thoughts. The goal is to make this routine a signal—a ritual that gently guides you toward rest.

Only lie down when you're actually sleepy. If you find yourself wide awake and staring at the ceiling, get up. Sit somewhere quiet and do something gentle like reading, breathing, or praying. Return to bed when your body feels ready. Over time, this helps rebuild a strong mental connection between your bed and actual sleep.

It takes time to build a new sleep rhythm. You might not feel the shift immediately, but your body is always listening. Keep showing up for rest, even when it feels elusive. You're reminding your nervous system what safety feels like. This isn't about perfection, it's about practice. Night after night, you're laying the foundation for a healthier, more resilient mind.

If sleep remains a struggle even after these changes—if you're dealing with persistent insomnia or restlessness, or are waking up exhausted—it might be worth exploring deeper issues like sleep apnea, chronic pain, or anxiety-related sleep disturbances. You don't have to figure it out alone. Speaking with a medical professional can provide clarity, solutions, and support.

Sleep is not an indulgence, it's infrastructure. It's the drain that clears emotional residue, repairs your nervous system, and gives you the strength to meet your day. Without it, your bucket fills faster and empties more slowly. Prioritize it like your mental health depends on it—because it does. And when you do, everything else starts to feel just a little more manageable.

The next section will explore how to carry the restoration of sleep into the rhythm of your waking hours—through intentional movement that supports both your body and mind.

Case Example:

Sarah had always considered herself adaptable—able to stay up late finishing work or scrolling on her phone, then bounce back the next day with a cup of coffee and a quick breakfast on the go. Her sleep schedule shifted constantly depending on the demands of the week. Late nights were common, and catch-up sleep on weekends became her routine. At first, it felt manageable. But over time, the cracks began to show. She noticed a steady drop in energy. Focus became harder to maintain, and her usual sharpness at work started to dull. To get through the day, she leaned on sugar, energy drinks, and frequent caffeine boosts. It was a short-term fix that led to long-term consequences—her cravings grew, her weight crept up, and she started to feel emotionally flat. When a close friend shared how a consistent sleep schedule had transformed her own health, Sarah was skeptical. How could something as simple as bedtime make that much of a difference? But curiosity and exhaustion won out. With her friend's support, she began experimenting—setting a fixed wake-up time, winding down with low lights and screen limits, and protecting her sleep window as if it were an important meeting. Within a week, she noticed a shift. Her mood steadied. Cravings eased. She wasn't dragging herself through the day anymore. Encouraged, she read more about sleep hygiene and refined her routine—gradually creating a system that worked for her life. Months later, Sarah felt like a different person. She no longer relied on sugar and caffeine to function. Her focus returned, her energy improved, and emotionally she felt more grounded. Sleep, once an afterthought, had quietly become the foundation for her physical and mental well-being.

6.3 Exercise

Your body was made to move. And when you give it that chance—even just a little—it doesn't just get stronger. Your mind gets lighter. Your thoughts get clearer. Your emotions settle. Exercise isn't only about shaping muscles or hitting a goal on a fitness tracker. It's one of the most effective ways to open the drain on your mental health bucket. When stress builds up, movement becomes a release. A reset. A quiet reminder that you're not stuck—you're still capable of change, even if it's just one step at a time.

It doesn't take much. Just 30 minutes of moderate movement a few times a week can shift the way your body and brain handle stress.[12] They all count: those walks around the block, a quick jog, a slow bike ride. One of the first things you might notice is how you sleep. Movement helps reset your internal clock, guiding your body into deeper, more restorative rest. And when sleep improves, everything else starts to feel more manageable.

Beyond rest, exercise builds endurance—not just physical stamina, but emotional stamina too.[13,14] You start showing up for your life with more energy and less fatigue. The little things feel a bit less heavy. You're able to take on more without immediately hitting a wall. Then there are the chemicals—the ones your brain naturally produces when you move: endorphins, dopamine, serotonin. These are your built-in mood lifters. They ease anxiety, brighten your outlook, and soften the edges of sadness or stress.

Regular movement doesn't just help you feel better in the moment—it rewires your brain over time.

You don't need to feel motivated to move. In fact, movement often creates motivation.[15] Some days you'll feel too tired, too tense, or too overwhelmed to start—but that's exactly when your body might need it most. Because movement doesn't just burn energy—it creates it.

When you exercise, blood flow increases throughout your brain, nourishing the areas that carry your emotional and cognitive load.[16,17,18] The limbic system—your emotional command center—gets a boost, helping stabilize mood and motivation. The amygdala, which deals with fear and stress, becomes less reactive. And the hippocampus, responsible for memory and learning, actually grows stronger. This means that regular movement doesn't just help you feel better in the moment—it rewires your brain over time. You build emotional flexibility. You learn to respond instead of react. You get better at bouncing back when life knocks you sideways.

You don't need to train for a marathon or hit the gym every day. You don't need fancy equipment or a rigid plan. What matters most is consistency and joy. Start small. A few minutes a day is enough to begin. Walk your dog a little farther. Stretch when you wake up. Try to treat movement like you would any important part of your day. Put it on your calendar. Keep a pair of shoes by the door. Make it easy to begin—even when your motivation is low.

Don't be afraid to switch things up—variety not only keeps exercise interesting but also gives your body and brain fresh challenges. One day, try yoga; the next, take a brisk walk. Swim, garden, stretch—whatever feels good. Some days you may prefer solitude, while other times moving alongside a friend can help you stay motivated. The best kind of exercise is the one you'll actually do—the one that feels energizing rather than punishing, and the one that fits into your life, not the other way around.

Movement is one of the most accessible and reliable tools for building mental resilience—it's always within reach, even on the hardest days (especially on those days). When your bucket feels full and heavy, exercise offers a gentle way to release some of that weight—not all at once, but gradually, through consistency, patience, and self-kindness.

It's more than a workout, it's a form of self-respect. A declaration to yourself that your well-being matters. That you're worth the effort. That even when life gets loud and messy, you still get to show up for yourself—one breath, one step, one stretch at a time.

The next section will explore how nourishment extends beyond movement, and how the quality of your food influences recovery, focus, and emotional balance.

6.4 Diet

What you eat doesn't just shape your body, it shapes your mind. Every bite, every snack, and every meal sends signals to your brain. Some of those signals can sharpen your focus, balance your mood, and build resilience. Others can do the opposite, leaving you with heaviness, brain fog, or unexplained fatigue. Your gut isn't just a digestive organ—it's a command center, often referred to as your "second brain." Inside your gastrointestinal tract are millions of nerve endings and trillions of bacteria, collectively called the microbiome. This vast, living ecosystem plays a central role in your mental health. It affects how you digest food, how strong your immune system is, and even how you feel emotionally.[19]

Your gut isn't just a digestive organ—it's a command center, often referred to as your "second brain."

Interestingly, about 90–95 percent of the body's serotonin is produced in the gastrointestinal tract, not the brain.[20] While this serotonin doesn't directly impact brain chemistry because of the blood-brain barrier, the gut still significantly influences mental health through the gut-brain axis. A healthy gut contributes to balanced inflammation, a thriving microbiota, and effective signaling pathways that help regulate mood, emotions, and cognitive clarity. But when your gut is inflamed, neglected, or overwhelmed with processed foods, everything becomes more difficult. Sleep suffers, energy crashes, emotional regulation falters, and even minor stress can feel overwhelming.

It's easy to overlook how food directly affects your mental state, but the connection is clear. Diets high in refined sugars, ultra-processed ingredients, and artificial additives are strongly linked to poorer mental health outcomes.[21] These foods can cause spikes in blood sugar and insulin, lead to systemic inflammation, and disrupt neurotransmitter balance. Over time, this biochemical disruption translates into emotional symptoms like irritability, mental fog, low motivation, and a general feeling of unease. Fortunately, there is a better path—one that doesn't rely on extreme dieting or guilt, but on awareness, intention, and nourishment.

Eating well doesn't just fuel your body, it helps open the drain on your mental stress bucket. When your brain is properly nourished, your energy remains stable, and your gut is functioning well, it becomes easier to manage tough days. You gain more emotional resilience, your reactions become less intense, and your ability to recover improves. Certain dietary patterns can even reduce the risk of depression and improve stress tolerance. For example, the Mediterranean diets are associated with a 42–73 percent lower risk of developing depressive symptoms compared to the standard Western diet in certain world regions.[22]

What makes these diets different is their emphasis on whole, unprocessed foods. They include generous amounts of colorful vegetables, fruits, legumes, whole grains, nuts, seeds, seafood, and fermented foods like yogurt. They also reduce added sugars, limit red meat, and avoid heavily processed snacks or fast food. These dietary choices support a healthy microbiome, reduce inflammation, and provide the essential nutrients—vitamins, minerals, and antioxidants—your brain needs to function well.[23]

You don't have to completely overhaul your diet to begin seeing benefits. Start by paying attention to how certain foods make you feel. Does your lunch leave you feeling energized, or does it make you sleepy and bloated? Do certain snacks trigger brain fog? Are your cravings worse when you're emotionally drained or sleep-deprived? Becoming aware of these patterns is the first step. Next, make small, manageable changes. Choose whole grain bread over white bread. Swap sugary drinks for water or tea. Add leafy greens to meals that usually lack color. Opt for a protein-rich breakfast instead of sugary cereals or pastries.

Even tiny adjustments—like including a handful of berries, a spoonful of yogurt, or a sprinkle of seeds—can begin to shift your gut health and improve your mood over time. The goal is to gain momentum, starting with small wins. It's about treating your body with kindness and giving it what it needs to thrive.

Your gut is constantly sending messages to your brain. What you feed it determines the tone of those messages—whether they're calming and supportive or agitating and disruptive. Food isn't just fuel. It's information. It's medicine. It's one of the most consistent ways you can support your mental health every single day. When your diet supports your brain, you're better equipped to handle stress. You bounce back faster. You feel more focused, grounded, and capable.

So the next time you're deciding what to eat—whether in front of your fridge or when scanning a menu—pause and ask yourself what your "second brain" really needs. With each thoughtful choice, you give yourself the opportunity to let go of what drains you and replenish yourself with what sustains you.

The next section will explore how substances like alcohol and cannabis can affect your mood, sleep, and stress response, sometimes helping in the short term but quietly undermining your mental health over time.

6.5 Substances: The "Clogs" That Impair Your Mental Health Drains

Even when everything else seems to be going well—solid sleep, regular exercise, improved diet—certain habits can quietly undermine your progress. Substances like alcohol and cannabis often offer the promise of comfort, but beneath the surface they frequently work against your healing. In the context of the Mental Health Bucket Model, they don't just fail to open the drains; they often clog them, making it harder for stress to leave your system. That's why paying attention to these substances is so important—not with judgment, but with honesty. If they're becoming regular tools to escape or self-soothe, they may be quietly undoing the recovery you're working so hard to build.

Alcohol often wears a friendly face. It's part of social gatherings, relaxation rituals, and celebrations. One drink to unwind, one glass to take the edge off seems harmless. But alcohol is a central nervous system depressant, and it changes brain chemistry in ways that may cause your stress bucket to overflow more quickly than you realize.[24] Initially, it slows things down and brings a sense of ease. But that calm is short-lived. As alcohol leaves your system, the brain often rebounds in the opposite direction, triggering increased stress signals that can make you feel more anxious, irritable, or emotionally fragile. This bounce-back effect is a real neurological response, not just your imagination, and it can create a cycle: Drink to feel better, feel worse when it wears off, and drink again to soothe the comedown.

Alcohol also affects sleep—even if it helps you fall asleep at first. It disrupts REM cycles and fragments your rest, leaving you tired, foggy, and more emotionally vulnerable the next day.[25] Because sleep is your most important drain, alcohol effectively corks it. Over time, alcohol can slowly unravel the emotional and mental stability you're trying to strengthen.

It interferes with memory, emotional regulation, and decision-making. It can widen cracks in relationships, diminish self-trust, and delay healing in ways that might not become obvious until much later. Even if your drinking doesn't meet the clinical definition of addiction, it may still be contributing more harm than benefit. If your nervous system feels stuck in a heightened state of alert, alcohol might be part of what's keeping it there.

Cannabis use is more complex than it may seem. For some individuals, it can feel like a lifeline, and is often used to manage anxiety, insomnia, pain, or appetite issues.[26,27] It can indeed provide short-term relief, but the long-term effects are far less predictable. The calming benefits tend to fade with regular use, leading many to increase their dose or frequency to achieve the same sense of ease. What may begin as occasional use can gradually evolve into a daily habit, especially when it appears to make everyday life more tolerable. Over time, however, side effects can accumulate—manifesting as rebound anxiety, memory lapses, difficulty concentrating, reduced motivation, and poor-quality sleep that leaves you feeling unrested.[28,29] For those with a personal or family history of mental illness, cannabis may worsen or even trigger symptoms such as paranoia or psychosis.[30] Even in less severe cases, it can subtly interfere with emotional regulation, leading to a sense of numbness, reduced mental clarity, and difficulty connecting with yourself and others.

It's easy to think, *But this helps me*. And maybe it does—at least in the short term. But if your emotional lows are becoming deeper, your mornings heavier, or your motivation weaker, these substances might be contributing more stress than they're relieving. If you've worked hard to improve your sleep, nutrition, and physical movement, it's worth asking whether these habits are quietly canceling out your progress.

This conversation isn't about shame—it's about clarity. If a substance that once brought comfort is now causing more harm than good, it's okay to want a different path. And if cutting back or quitting feels intimidating, you don't have to do it alone. Medical professionals, therapists, and supportive communities can help you find new ways that nurture your peace rather than postpone your pain. Removing these clogs—one shift at a time—makes room for real healing to take root. It keeps your drains open and allows your nervous system to breathe again. Sometimes true recovery doesn't come from adding something new but from releasing what quietly holds you back.

While substances can change how you feel from the outside in, mindfulness works from the inside out. In the next section, you'll learn how this practice helps regulate your stress response and rebuild resilience.

Case Example:

Mike never thought much about his drinking. It started off simple—celebrations, weekend gatherings, dinner with friends. A few drinks here and there to mark the moment. He enjoyed being social, and alcohol felt like a natural part of it all. But slowly the pattern changed. Weekends turned into weekdays. Drinking shifted from something shared to something solitary. Before long, it became part of his nightly routine—his way to unwind after a long day, to quiet his mind before sleep. At first, it seemed harmless. But then he began to notice the aftereffects. His mornings felt sluggish. His mood grew unpredictable. He needed caffeine to stay alert and sugar to boost his energy. His sleep became shallow, and the energy he once brought to work and social settings started to fade. He was less focused, more irritable, and no longer as engaged in the relationships that mattered most. His close friends noticed too. After a difficult but honest conversation, Mike agreed to take a closer look at his habits. It took time to move from defensiveness to acceptance, but eventually he reached out for help. With support, he started to cut back. He learned new ways to manage stress—walks, journaling, calling a friend instead of reaching for a drink. He restructured his social life around activities that didn't revolve around alcohol. Gradually, his clarity returned. So did his sleep, his energy, and his ability to show up more fully in his life. Mike didn't need to hit rock bottom to realize something was off. He just needed to recognize that what once felt like relief had quietly become a barrier. And by stepping back, he found more of himself than he expected to recover.

6.6 Mindfulness: The Mental Drain That Grounds You in the Present

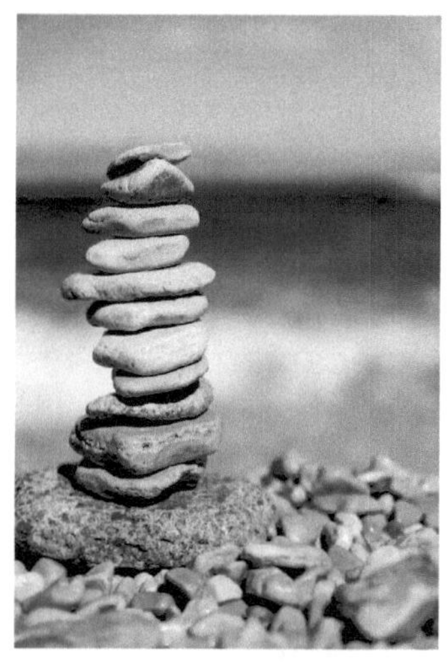

Some drains are physical—you sleep, move, eat well, and feel better. But others work beneath the surface. They are quiet and subtle. Mindfulness is one of those. It's not about doing more, it's about noticing what's already happening. It's about being where your feet are, rather than chasing thoughts that pull you away. You live in a world that makes it easy to disconnect from the moment. Notifications, deadlines, conversations, traffic, and timelines all pull your attention in five directions at once. And with that constant pull, your mental health bucket starts to fill—not always in dramatic splashes but often in small, invisible drips. One anxious thought, one frustrating exchange, one scary headline, or one regret looping on repeat can each contribute to the overflow. Mindfulness helps open a drain—not by changing your life overnight, but by changing your relationship to it, one breath, one moment, one thought at a time.

Mindfulness means being aware of the present moment without judging it. It's not about trying to escape it, fix it, or run from it. It's about staying with it. It is the skill of noticing your thoughts and feelings without letting them carry you away. You've likely experienced mindful moments without realizing it—watching your child sleep, drinking tea on a quiet morning, or listening to nature and feeling completely present. In those moments, the past fades, the future pauses, and you're fully in the now. Mindfulness is about learning to create more of those moments deliberately. It requires willingness and a simple decision to pause, to pay attention, and to return again and again to the only place your life is actually happening—the present.

Mindfulness helps open a drain—not by changing your life overnight, but by changing your relationship to it, one breath, one moment, one thought at a time.

Your nervous system reacts to perceived threats, whether real or imagined. An email from your boss, a memory from 10 years ago, or a fear about next week can all trigger stress. Your body doesn't always know the difference. It reacts with a racing heart, tight chest, and shallow breath. The stress faucet turns on. Mindfulness doesn't eliminate life's stressors, but it helps regulate your response. It creates space between stimulus and reaction. Instead of spiraling into panic, you pause. Instead of being swept away by anger or fear, you observe it. This pause is powerful. It lowers cortisol, slows your heart rate, and activates the parasympathetic nervous system.[31,32] It signals to your body: *You're safe right now.* And when your body feels safe, your bucket starts draining.

Mindfulness also impacts the brain. It strengthens the prefrontal cortex, which is responsible for awareness, focus, and self-regulation, and it quiets the amygdala, which governs fear and emotional reactivity.[33,34] With regular practice, the brain becomes less reactive and more resilient. In essence, you're rewiring your internal system—not to prevent stress entirely but to keep it from owning you. Over time, mindfulness builds emotional regulation, lowers anxiety, improves sleep, and enhances attention. These aren't just feel-good outcomes; they are measurable, biological changes that contribute to a stronger, calmer version of you.

Mindfulness isn't always about sitting in meditation. Sometimes it shows up in tiny, barely noticeable moments—like taking a deep breath before answering a tough question, feeling the weight of your body in a chair instead of numbing with your phone, or noticing that you're overwhelmed and stepping outside for fresh air. It might be observing a judgmental thought and choosing not to follow it. It can be brushing your teeth and actually feeling the bristles, eating without looking at a screen and tasting your food, performing your religious rituals or prayers, or hearing your child laugh and letting that be enough. You don't need an app or a yoga mat. You need presence. Just five mindful minutes a day is enough to begin. Over time, those minutes stretch, and mindfulness becomes less of a practice and more of a way of being.

If you're not sure where to begin, there are a few accessible techniques you can try:[35,36,37]

1. Breath awareness: Close your eyes and bring your attention to your breath. Notice the inhale. Notice the exhale. When your mind wanders—and it will—gently bring it back.
2. Body scan: Lie down or sit comfortably, then move your attention through your body from head to toe, noticing where tension hides and what feels open or heavy.
3. Mindful walking: Leave your phone behind and walk slowly, feeling the ground under your feet, listening to the wind, and paying attention to your posture.
4. Thought labeling: When a strong thought or emotion arises, name it: "This is anger," "This is worry," or "This is judgment." Naming provides distance and reminds you that you are not your thoughts.
5. Finally, the 5-4-3-2-1 grounding technique can return you to the moment when you feel overwhelmed: Name five things you see, four you can touch, three you can hear, two you can smell, and one you can taste.

When you begin a mindfulness practice, you may notice feelings of distraction or restlessness. That's a normal part of the process. The goal isn't to clear your mind completely but to practice returning your focus. Each time you bring your attention back, you are strengthening a mental muscle. It is the act of returning that truly matters. On some days, you may feel more grounded and present. On other days, you may struggle to focus at all. The key is to continue showing up regardless of how you feel. There is no pressure to perform and no need for expectations—just the intention to pay attention. Think of mindfulness like brushing your mental teeth: You are not doing it to be perfect but to stay clear and maintain mental hygiene.

Mindfulness won't erase your stress, but it changes your relationship to it. It helps you respond with intention rather than react with panic. It helps you notice what's real instead of being hijacked by what's imagined. Most of all, it helps you feel like yourself again—not some perfect version, just the version that's present, steady, and aware. You don't have to master it. You just have to begin.

Eventually, mindfulness becomes more than something you practice; it becomes something you live. You start catching yourself before snapping. You hear your thoughts before believing them. You pause before reacting. That's the change. It becomes a reflex—a drain that stays open without effort. A way of being present in your own life instead of drifting through it.

Mindfulness is quiet work. There is no loud transformation or instant result. But over time, it builds a foundation. It turns down the volume on the mental noise and makes space for clarity and peace. You deserve that space. You deserve the calm that comes from being rooted in the now. And now it's time to look at how to keep these drains working—not just when you're feeling good but when you're stressed, tired, or overwhelmed.

Mindfulness is quiet work. There is no loud transformation or instant result. But over time, it builds a foundation.

The next section will explore how habits are built, how they're broken, and how to make the things that help you feel better stick for the long haul.

6.7 Building Lasting Habits

Understanding the importance of sleep, movement, mindfulness, nutrition, and minimizing harmful substances is a strong foundation for mental wellness. But understanding alone rarely guarantees action. You may already know that going for a walk, eating more vegetables, or putting your phone away before bed would help you feel better. Yet knowing what's good for you and consistently doing it are two very different things. That space between knowledge and action is where many people falter—not because they lack motivation but because they lack systems. This is where habits come in. Habits remove the burden of constant decision-making. They shift helpful behaviors from something you have to push yourself to do into something you simply do as part of your daily rhythm. Over time, they turn mental health practices from chores into something closer to reflex.

The goal isn't to follow every routine flawlessly. It's to return to them consistently enough that they become part of your identity—even on days when you're exhausted, overwhelmed, or distracted. When those supportive behaviors become integrated into your life, your drains stay open. You stop waiting until your bucket is overflowing to take care of yourself. Instead, you create steady release valves that help you manage stress before it builds to a breaking point. True resilience isn't about reacting at the edge of burnout—it's about having structures in place that prevent you from getting there.

At its core, a habit is simply a behavior that's repeated often enough in a similar context that it becomes automatic.[38,39,40] Most habits follow a predictable pattern: a cue, followed by a routine, and then a reward. For example, the cue might be waking up in the morning. The routine could be doing five minutes of light stretching. The reward is that you feel more alert and centered. When this cycle repeats regularly, your brain starts to anticipate the benefit and nudges you to follow through, often without the internal negotiation you used to need.

Creating lasting habits doesn't require brute force or endless motivation. It requires design and consistency. One of the most effective strategies is starting small—so small that it feels almost effortless.[41] Instead of deciding you'll meditate for 30 minutes each morning, start with 2. Instead of vowing to overhaul your diet, begin by adding a handful of greens to one meal a day. These tiny wins build momentum, and that momentum reinforces consistency. Small steps remove the friction that often derails bigger goals, making it more likely that you'll follow through even on tough days. And consistency, more than intensity, is what creates lasting change.

Another way to strengthen a habit is to attach it to something you already do. These "habit anchors" are actions you perform regularly—brushing your teeth, pouring coffee, walking the dog. They become cues for your new routine. If you want to practice gratitude, write down one thing you're thankful for right after brushing your teeth. If you want to move more, do a few stretches while waiting for your morning coffee to brew. These connections help embed your new behavior into your existing rhythm, reducing the mental effort required to begin.

Environment plays a major role too. Your surroundings shape your behavior far more than most people realize. If unhealthy snacks are the first thing you see in your pantry, they become the default. If your meditation cushion is tucked away in a closet, you're less likely to use it. Design your space with your goals in mind. Leave your water bottle where it's visible. Place your journal on your nightstand. Charge your phone outside your bedroom if you want to improve sleep. When your environment aligns with your intentions, supportive habits become easier to maintain.

Of course, even with the best systems, life doesn't always cooperate. You'll have days where you're too tired, busy, or emotionally drained to complete your full routine. That's why it helps to plan for imperfection. Create a "minimum version" of each habit—a scaled-down fallback that you can do even when your day falls apart. Instead of skipping your workout entirely, take a five-minute walk. Instead of journaling a full page, write a single sentence. These smaller acts keep the habit alive and maintain the sense of continuity. Missing one day isn't the problem—it's letting one day become a week or a month. Having a backup plan keeps your progress intact.

Tracking your efforts can also strengthen your commitment.[42,43] It doesn't have to be elaborate. A checkmark on a calendar, a line in a notebook, or an app on your phone can all help you see your progress in real time. More importantly, take a moment to acknowledge how each action makes you feel. Recognizing the benefit reinforces your motivation. Let the feeling of a clear mind after a walk or a calmer body after deep breathing settle in. That emotional feedback helps rewire the habit loop and makes you more likely to return to it.

Community support can make habits more sustainable too. Sharing your goals with someone else—whether it's a partner, friend, or group—creates a sense of accountability. Knowing someone else is working toward similar changes or cheering you on can help you stay engaged on days when your own motivation wavers. You don't have to go it alone. Even one conversation about your habit goals can bring clarity and encouragement.

And when setbacks happen—and they will—respond with self-compassion, not self-criticism. Missing a day doesn't erase your progress. It doesn't mean you've failed. It simply means you're human. What matters most is what you do next. Be gentle. Return to your routine. Think of your habits like a path through the woods. Sometimes you step off. But you always know the way back.

Long-lasting change takes time. Habits aren't formed overnight, and they aren't maintained through intensity alone. They grow through quiet repetition—through showing up, again and again, even when it's inconvenient or imperfect. Over time, the behaviors that once felt effortful become part of how you move through the world. You'll find yourself choosing what supports you, not because you're forcing it but because it's become your norm.

You don't need to fix everything at once. Choose one area to focus on—whether it's sleep, nutrition, movement, or mindfulness. Start where it feels doable. Keep it simple. Keep it consistent. With patience and persistence, your habits will form a safety net—one that helps keep your bucket from overflowing and supports you in becoming more resilient, grounded, and healthy.

In the next section, the focus shifts from personal habits to interpersonal healing—exploring how connection with others can strengthen your capacity to cope, heal, and thrive.

Case Example:

Daisy had always admired the benefits of exercise. She read books on it, followed fitness influencers, and knew the science behind how movement improves mood, metabolism, focus, and long-term health. On paper, she was more than prepared. She didn't lack motivation or knowledge—she genuinely wanted exercise to be a regular part of her life. And yet every time she started a routine, it fizzled out within weeks. It wasn't about choosing the wrong workout. She had tried yoga, running, HIIT, strength training—all with enthusiasm. But life would inevitably get in the way. A few late nights at work, travel plans, unexpected errands, and the momentum vanished. Each time it happened, Daisy felt discouraged and puzzled. Why was something she believed in so hard to maintain? That's when a friend introduced her to the science of habit formation. Daisy shifted her focus from "what" to "how." She began learning about cues, routines, and rewards. She realized that habits weren't just about willpower—they were about systems. She studied how friction can derail a good intention, and how small tweaks—like laying out workout clothes the night before or setting a recurring calendar alert—can make all the difference. She also learned the importance of flexibility. Instead of rigid expectations, she created a menu of workout options: short walks for busy days, virtual classes for rainy days, strength sessions when she had more time. Crucially, she stopped waiting for motivation and started relying on structure. She built micro-routines around her workouts—like drinking water first thing in the morning or listening to a favorite podcast—to create a rhythm that felt natural. Progress wasn't instant, but it was steady. Eventually exercise stopped feeling like a task to check off and started becoming part of who she was. She didn't need to force it anymore—it simply fit. Other priorities began to align around it, rather than the other way around. Daisy's story shows that the gap between knowing and doing is often bridged not by effort alone but by thoughtful design. Once she learned how habits really work, she didn't just work out—she became someone who moves, consistently, with joy and intention.

6.8 The Social Connection: It Takes a Village

You've already taken on a lot. You've begun noticing the stress that fills your mental health bucket. You've become more aware of how your nervous system responds and started examining the roles that sleep, movement, nutrition, and even substance use play in your well-being. You've explored what it takes to turn these insights into consistent habits. But even with all that progress, there's a truth that often gets overlooked: You can be doing everything "right" and still feel overwhelmed. That feeling doesn't mean you're failing—it means you were never designed to handle everything on your own.

Human beings are wired for connection, not as a bonus but as a biological necessity.[44,45] You need other people—not just for joy and laughter or celebrating milestones but to help share the emotional weight of everyday life. And that weight adds up more often than most people are willing to admit. Your closest relationships can act like external drains for your bucket. These are the people who can sit with you when your thoughts feel tangled, who notice when something's off before you've even said a word, and who remind you of your strength when you forget you have any left. They serve as mirrors, as anchors, and as gentle pressure valves that release what might otherwise build silently inside.

Human beings are wired for connection, not as a bonus but as a biological necessity.

You've likely experienced this—even in subtle moments—such as the relief that comes after venting to a trusted friend or the noticeable shift in your body when someone listens with full presence, without interrupting, trying to fix, or passing judgment. Alternatively, it may have been a long time since you've felt genuinely seen, and the idea of opening up to someone might feel uncomfortable or uncertain. That is perfectly understandable. However, regardless of where you are starting from, one truth remains constant: Connection is not a weakness, it is a fundamental part of being human. Repeated studies confirm what our instincts already tell us—meaningful relationships help buffer against burnout, protect physical health, and enhance our ability to adapt to change.[46,47] Individuals with strong social support systems tend to recover more quickly, cope more effectively, and live longer.[48,49] Still, being around others is not enough on its own. What matters most is the depth and quality of those connections.

You can be married, surrounded by coworkers, even admired—and still feel isolated. That's because what truly sustains us is not mere presence, but presence that comes with depth, trust, and safety. The kind of relationship where it feels okay to show up as your full self, not just your filtered or polished version. So take a moment to reflect: Who in your life fits that description? Who has seen you at your most vulnerable and stayed close? Who do you feel comfortable calling when you're anxious, exhausted, or just not okay?

If no one immediately comes to mind, you're not alone. Many people feel this absence—especially in adulthood, when connection requires more deliberate effort. But just because these people aren't currently in your life doesn't mean they can't be. They may be waiting to be rediscovered or newly formed. Maybe there's someone you've drifted from—not due to conflict but from the wear and tear of daily life. Maybe there's someone you already spend time with but haven't truly opened up to. Or maybe it's time to build new bridges—through a community group, a spiritual space, a book club, a shared hobby, or a mental health support network.

Your village doesn't need to be large. It only needs to be real. One or two people who offer genuine support can make a world of difference. Not because they'll solve your problems but because they'll help you carry them. That kind of shared emotional load can be the difference between feeling like you're barely holding on and feeling held.[50,51]

And don't forget that your role in relationships isn't just to receive support—you also have the power to offer it. Sometimes the act of showing up for others is what helps ground us in our own healing. A thoughtful message, a listening ear, a check-in at the right moment—these are not small things. They are lifelines. When support flows both ways, trust deepens and resilience expands.

You don't need to wait for a crisis to reach out. Invest in connection now. Nurture the relationships that already exist. Make space for new ones to grow. Check in before you think it's needed. Follow up on things people mentioned in passing. Allow conversations to go deeper than surface-level updates. Be willing to share something real, even if it feels vulnerable. And when someone entrusts you with their truth, meet it with care, patience, and presence. Listen more than you speak. Ask what they need. Be a safe place for someone to land.

While stress is part of being human, isolation doesn't have to be. You're not weak for needing others—you're wise for seeking support. And when your own strength feels depleted, it's often the strength of your relationships that keeps you steady. Think of your support system as the final and most often overlooked drain in your mental health bucket model. It won't show up on a checklist or a chart, but it might just be the most vital of them all.

So tend to your connections. Reach out with intention. Deepen what's already present, and stay open to what's possible. Because in the end, resilience isn't built alone. It's built through the hands that hold us when our bucket is full—and the presence of people who help lighten the load.

6.9 Drains: Takeaways and Management Strategies

After exploring what fills your mental health bucket—those constant inputs of pressure, demands, and emotional weight—it becomes impossible to ignore how critical your drains really are. These aren't just wellness trends or self-help clichés. They are the essential, often overlooked systems that keep you grounded, functioning, and able to return to yourself. Drains matter because they create space. When they work well, they allow you to release what doesn't belong inside you: tension, noise, and overwhelm. Practices like sleep, movement, nutrition, mindfulness, and setting boundaries around substances aren't just ways to "feel better." They're the daily mechanisms that prevent you from drowning in everything life pours in.

When these drains are neglected, the opposite happens. You may start to feel more fragile, less tolerant, and less motivated. Tasks that once felt manageable can suddenly become overwhelming. This is what happens when the bucket fills faster than it can drain. The good news is that you have influence over these drains. You don't need to overhaul your entire life in a weekend. You just need to start tending to the systems that help you let go. Begin where you are, using what you already have. Often the smallest shifts are the most powerful.

You've already taken the time to understand the core drains that support mental resilience. Sleep acts as your reset button; when you prioritize rest, everything improves—memory, mood, clarity, and immunity. If sleep is off, your whole system struggles to recover. Exercise isn't just about physical strength—it also helps clear emotional residue. A brisk walk, a few stretches, or swimming a few laps can release cortisol, process adrenaline, and help your nervous system return to baseline. Your diet fuels more than just your body; it influences brain chemistry. A nourished body leads to a more stable mind. When inflammation, blood sugar crashes, or poor gut health are present, your mood, energy, and clarity suffer.

Substance use can either support or hinder your well-being. While alcohol, cannabis, or other substances might offer temporary relief, they often do so by numbing rather than healing. Overuse can cloud the very drains you're trying to open. Mindfulness helps bring you back to the present moment. It isn't about detaching from life—it's about slowing down, reducing the mental static, and creating a pause between stimulus and reaction. Habit formation helps transform all of these practices from conscious effort into second nature. What you repeat consistently rewires your brain, and once a behavior becomes a habit, it no longer requires the same level of decision-making or willpower. Lastly, social connection is often the most overlooked yet powerful drain. Feeling seen, supported, and understood allows the nervous system to relax in a way that solo efforts can't replicate. You don't need a wide social circle—just a few real, trustworthy relationships that allow you to exhale and remember your worth.

Ultimately, drains aren't about escaping stress but learning how to process it—so it doesn't accumulate, weigh you down, or take control of your life. When your drains are functioning, you don't just feel better—you respond more thoughtfully, recover more quickly, and navigate difficulties with greater strength. These practices don't eliminate struggle, but they create the inner space to hold it with more stability. And when your drains work, your bucket doesn't spill—not because stress disappears but because you've built a reliable system that allows it to release.

This system isn't built through grand gestures. It's built through small, consistent decisions that stack up over time. It's the five minutes of breathwork you take in the morning, the walk you squeeze in after lunch, the phone call to a friend, or the decision to skip a drink and go to bed early. These moments might seem insignificant on their own, but collectively they are everything. This is how real recovery happens—not all at once but through one thoughtful moment, one intentional action, and one cleared drain at a time.

The Habit Formation Exercise: Strengthening Your Drains

You've now seen that your drains—sleep, movement, nutrition, mindfulness, substance boundaries, and social connection—aren't luxuries. They're essential release valves that keep your mental health bucket from overflowing. But drains only work when they're maintained. That's where habit formation comes in. In engineering terms, this is preventive maintenance: small, routine actions that prevent system failure. In psychological terms, it's behavioral conditioning—the process of wiring healthy responses until they run automatically, with less resistance and more ease.

This exercise will help you identify the most critical drains that need enhancement or reinforcement, and then use a proven framework—cue, action, reward, environment, and coupling—to turn intention into lasting habit.

Step 1: Identify Your Top Three Drains

Look over the areas you've just explored: sleep and rest, physical activity, nutrition and hydration, mindfulness and self-reflection, limiting or managing substances, and building social connection. Ask yourself: Which of these, if strengthened, would make the biggest difference right now? Circle or write down your top three drains to focus on over the next few weeks. These are not just areas to "improve." They are systems to reinforce—so your bucket can release pressure naturally, even on the hardest days.

Step 2: Define Your Target Habit for Each Drain

For each of your top three drains, write a single small, concrete habit you'd like to build. Instead of "sleep more," try "turn off screens 30 minutes before bed." Instead of "exercise more," try "stretch for five minutes after work." Instead of "eat better," try "pack a balanced lunch the night before." Keep it small. Sustainable habits are built through repetition, not intensity.

Step 3: Use the Habit Formation Framework

For each chosen habit, fill in the following five prompts:

1. Cue: What will remind you to do it? (e.g., alarm, time of day, visual cue, or routine anchor)
2. Action: What specific behavior will you perform? (Make it measurable and short.)
3. Reward: What immediate benefit will you notice or celebrate? (Even a simple acknowledgment counts.)
4. Environment: What can you change around you to make this easier? (Lay out clothes, prep food, clear distractions.)
5. Habit Coupling: What existing routine can this new habit attach to? (e.g., after brushing your teeth, during your lunch break, before starting your commute)

Here's an example:

Drain: Sleep

1. Cue: 9:30 p.m. phone reminder to "power down."
2. Action: Turn off screens and read for 15 minutes.
3. Reward: Notice calmer breathing and lighter mood before bed.
4. Environment: Dim lights, move phone to another room.
5. Habit Coupling: Do this right after setting out clothes for tomorrow.

Step 4: Track and Adjust

Commit to practicing each habit for two weeks. At the end of each week, reflect: *Did I follow through consistently? What got in the way? What small adjustment would make this easier next time?* This process isn't about perfection. It's about engineering reliability—building self-care systems that work even when motivation fades.

Step 5: Revisit and Reinforce

After two to three weeks, reevaluate. Have any of these actions started to feel automatic? If so, that's your brain rewiring itself for sustainability. When one habit becomes routine, consider adding a second layer—another small change to strengthen that same drain or open a new one.

When you strengthen your drains through habit, you're not just adding wellness activities—you're upgrading your system's ability to *release pressure continuously*. Each small act compounds over time. The goal isn't to create a perfect routine. It's to make your healing predictable.

Visit TheBucketModel.com for a free printable download of this exercise and more.

Case Study: Rebuilding the Drains—A Young Man's Journey Toward Restoration

Ethan was in his mid-20s when things began to lose color. There wasn't a crisis or a dramatic unraveling—just a quiet, persistent dullness that settled into the rhythm of his life. He described it as a kind of fog, not thick enough to stop him in his tracks, but heavy enough to make everything feel like a drag. Days blurred together.

Energy ran low. Sleep became irregular, and mornings felt more like something to survive than a fresh start. He couldn't remember the last time something genuinely excited him. When asked what brought him joy or meaning, he went silent—not because he didn't want to answer but because he simply didn't know.

Ethan's routine lacked structure. Nights stretched out with screen time and substance use—alcohol to unwind, cannabis to numb. Some nights he overslept; others he stayed up until dawn. There was no rhythm, only reaction. His body rarely moved, and most of his social interaction took place through a screen. He scrolled, clicked, liked. But real connection rarely surfaced. Eventually, a family member noticed something was off. There wasn't a big confrontation—just a quiet concern and a gentle suggestion to talk to someone. Ethan agreed, more out of curiosity than any real belief it would help. But during his first mental health assessment, something stood out. There wasn't a glaring trauma or a catastrophic event. What emerged instead was absence—a long, slow erosion of the habits that support well-being. His mental health bucket wasn't overflowing, it was stagnating. There weren't enough drains.

Rather than rushing into a diagnosis, his clinician started with the basics—small, manageable steps focused on rebuilding his foundation. Nothing overwhelming. No expectation to change everything overnight. Just slow, intentional restoration. They began with sleep. It became the first pillar of his recovery. There were no complicated rules—just a regular wake-up time, a calming wind-down routine in the evening, and fewer screens after dark. At first it felt awkward. Ethan wasn't used to structure. But over time the morning fog began to lift. That one small shift gave him something he hadn't had in a long time: a starting point.

Movement came next. There was no pressure to join a gym or follow a rigorous plan—just walking outside, in fresh air. The combination of nature and movement brought small flickers of clarity. His body began to feel more alive. The act of putting one foot in front of the other became its own kind of therapy—not to escape life but to reenter it, one step at a time. As his energy returned, attention turned to the substances. Alcohol and cannabis had become companions, habits that filled the silence. But now, with support, he began asking harder questions: What was he trying to avoid? What could he do instead? Slowly, the patterns began to loosen. He started replacing old rituals with new ones—breathwork, drawing, evening calls with a friend he had drifted from.

Eventually, a bigger question came into focus: What was missing from his life? Not just what was wrong, but what was absent. With guidance, Ethan began exploring short-term goals and longer-term hopes—not framed as pressure but as possibility. Purpose didn't need to be dramatic or grand. It could begin quietly. He started noticing what felt meaningful to pursue—what actually felt like him. Those tiny changes began to build. His posture shifted. His tone of voice grew more grounded. His days started to feel lived rather than endured. The fog didn't disappear all at once, but something real began to return—his energy, his curiosity, his voice.

Ethan didn't need to transform everything. He needed to restore the basics—the drains that allow the mind and body to recover. What nearly unraveled him wasn't the intensity of his stress but the absence of outlets. Without sleep, movement, connection, and clarity, even minor challenges became too much to bear. This wasn't a story about one big breakthrough. It was a story of slowly bringing life back online. One night of better rest.

One walk. One honest conversation. One fewer drink. One mindful breath.

Ethan's story is a powerful reminder that mental health isn't only about fixing what's wrong—it's often about restoring what's been missing. When the inputs into your bucket feel too heavy, it's easy to focus on what's broken. But sometimes the issue isn't damage, it's depletion. Ethan didn't drown in trauma. He was slowly sinking in emptiness. And the way out wasn't an overhaul. It was the quiet act of noticing where he could begin to release pressure. His recovery started with the simple but profound: sleep, movement, awareness around substance use, and mindful connection. These weren't indulgences—they were lifelines.

If life has been feeling flat, foggy, or unusually heavy, it's worth asking: What drains might be blocked? What practices or rhythms used to help you feel alive and grounded—and when did they begin to fade away? Rebuilding your mental health doesn't have to begin with solving everything. It can begin by restoring space. Because sometimes healing begins not by fixing the problem but by making room for life to flow again.

Key Takeaway:

Ethan's story shows that burnout and emotional exhaustion don't always erupt from chaos—they often grow quietly in the absence of healthy outlets. His life didn't collapse under pressure, it dulled under neglect. When the drains that sustain mental health—sleep, movement, connection, and meaningful rhythm—fall away, even ordinary stress becomes too heavy to hold.

His recovery reminds us that healing doesn't always require radical change. It often begins with the basics: consistent rest, gentle movement, mindful awareness, and real human connection. These simple practices restore the body's rhythm and the mind's capacity to breathe again.

Ethan's transformation wasn't about chasing motivation or waiting for inspiration—it was about rebuilding function, one drain at a time. By tending to the neglected systems that allow release and renewal, he created space for vitality to return naturally. The lesson is clear: When life feels stagnant, don't look for more to do. Look for where the flow stopped, and start there.

Conclusion

By now it's clear that mental wellness isn't a fixed trait or a simple diagnosis. It's not something you're either doing right or wrong. It's a dynamic system shaped by your biology, your habits, your environment, and your past. And like any system, it needs maintenance, attention, and care. The Mental Health Bucket Model offers a way to finally make sense of why things feel so overwhelming sometimes—why exhaustion can feel bone-deep, why focus disappears, why anxiety surges even when nothing obvious is wrong, and, most importantly, what to do about it. This isn't just a framework, it's a mirror and a tool. It helps you see where your system is overloaded, where the pressure is coming from, and where the release valves need support. More than anything, it provides a map for understanding and healing burnout.

Picture your mental health as a bucket. Life pours into it constantly—deadlines, family responsibilities, health scares, inner criticism, global uncertainty, digital noise. These inputs, whether big or small, accumulate quickly. When too much flows in and not enough flows out, the bucket overflows. That overflow is what we call burnout. Burnout isn't just being tired. It's a signal that your system is saturated. It means your usual coping strategies aren't keeping up, and your energy, attention, and emotional flexibility are being depleted faster than they can recover. The early signs can be easy to overlook—irritability, brain fog, forgetfulness, and disconnection—but when they persist, the body eventually keeps the score.

Your bucket's size—the amount of stress you can carry before breaking down—isn't a measure of moral strength. It's shaped by biology, psychology, and life experience. Things like vitamin levels, hormone balance, trauma history, family dynamics, chronic illness, and past coping strategies all play a role. Some people have wider buckets; others have more fragile ones. The important thing is knowing your own and respecting it rather than resenting it or trying to match someone else's. Honoring your capacity is the first step toward sustainable mental health. That capacity can grow, but not if it's constantly ignored, pushed, or shamed.

Stress doesn't always arrive with flashing lights. Sometimes it shows up quietly through background worry, endless emails, or social comparison.

Stress doesn't always arrive with flashing lights. Sometimes it shows up quietly through background worry, endless emails, or social comparison. Other times it floods in with force, like during loss, conflict, or illness. Every one of these inputs is a faucet. Some pour quickly, others drip slowly, but all of them contribute to the rising water in your bucket. While not all faucets can be shut off, becoming aware of which ones are in your control allows you to make informed choices. You can start to ask whether you're overwhelmed because of what's happening or because of how much you're absorbing without release. Modern faucets, like constant news and social media, rarely stop on their own. They fill your bucket even when you think you're resting. That's why awareness matters first—and boundaries must follow.

Drains are what keep you from drowning. They aren't rewards for enduring the day, they're the systems that prevent the day from crushing you. Sleep clears mental clutter, resets your mood, and gives your brain a chance to heal. Exercise moves stress chemicals out of your system and replaces them with clarity and calm. Food doesn't just power your body, it stabilizes your emotions. Boundaries around substances prevent you from dulling the internal signals that tell you when something needs to change. Mindfulness creates breathing room so you can respond instead of react. Habits turn helpful choices into automatic ones, removing the burden of constant decision-making. Social connection reminds you that you are not alone in carrying life's weight. None of these are indulgences. They are essential. And the more you strengthen them, the more pressure your system can handle without burning out.

You can't recover from chronic stress with a single weekend off. One therapy session won't drain a bucket that's been overflowing for months. True recovery comes through repetition—through daily habits that remind your nervous system it's safe to let go. This is why building habits matters more than relying on willpower. Sustainable change starts with small, intentional shifts. Link new habits to existing ones. Track your progress. Celebrate small wins. Protect your recovery time as if your health depends on it—because often it does. Even the smallest consistent drain does more good than the biggest change you never maintain.

Burnout is not a sign of weakness. It's what happens when a strong system is pushed too hard for too long without enough relief. It's not a personal flaw. It's a mismatch between what's being asked of you and what your system can currently sustain. This model isn't about eliminating stress entirely; it gives you something even more valuable: clarity, language, and practical tools. It helps you understand the weight you're carrying and how to create space within it. It shifts your perspective from self-blame to self-awareness, from shame to strategy, and from barely surviving to gradually recovering.

This is not the end of the journey. It's a new way of walking through life. Every time you notice what's filling your bucket, you regain a measure of control. Every time you clear even a small drain, you lower your risk of burnout. Each boundary you set, each breath you take, each consistent habit you build is a step toward resilience. The question now is simple, yet powerful: Which faucet will you dial down? Which drain will you open today? You don't have to fix everything. You just need to begin clearing space—one drop at a time. This is how healing begins. Not by pushing harder but by creating the room to breathe again.

Appendix: The Mental Health Bucket Model Reflection Series

Overview

This guided reflection series is designed to accompany your journey through *Burnout: Where the Head Goes, the Body Follows*. Each worksheet builds upon the Mental Health Bucket Model framework—helping you understand, measure, and balance the interconnected forces that shape your mental health capacity.

Together, these three exercises form a structured system for insight and action:

1. **Bucket Size / Strengths, Weaknesses, Opportunities, and Threats (SWOT) Analysis**

   Explore the foundations of your capacity.

   Identify internal strengths and vulnerabilities, as well as external opportunities and threats that influence your ability to manage stress and recover.
2. **Input Mapping Worksheet**

   Understand what pours into your bucket.

   Map your main sources of stress by volume, frequency, and controllability. Awareness of your inputs allows for strategic boundaries and intentional adjustments.

3. **Drains Habit Tracker**

   Strengthen your release systems.

   Build sustainable habits around rest, movement, nutrition, mindfulness, and connection. Learn to automate recovery through consistent, small actions.

How to Use This Series

- Complete each exercise after finishing its corresponding section in the book.
- Use them as living documents—revisit and update them as your circumstances and insights evolve.
- Reflect honestly. The purpose isn't perfection; it's awareness and progress.

A Note from the Author

These reflections are meant to bring the engineering mindset into emotional healing—to give structure to what often feels intangible. Every system can be understood, adjusted, and improved. Your mind and body are no different.

Approach these pages not as homework but as maintenance—an act of care for the system that is you.

For a free printable version of these worksheets and additional resources, visit TheBucketModel.com.

Bucket Size SWOT Exercise

Purpose: To help you analyze the core factors that shape your mental health capacity (your bucket size) through the lens of a SWOT analysis—an engineering and leadership tool for understanding systems and making strategic improvements.

Step 1: Define Your Context

Before you begin, take a moment to recall what influences the size of your mental health bucket—genetics, temperament, health conditions, trauma, environment, and social supports. These are the variables that determine how much stress you can hold and how you recover.

Step 2: Map Your SWOT

Use the table below to explore your internal and external factors. Be honest and specific. This isn't a test of strength—it's a map of reality.

Category	**Description**	**Examples**
Strengths	Internal traits or resources that enhance your resilience and expand your capacity	Supportive relationships, physical health, therapy engagement, problem-solving skills, sense of purpose
Weaknesses	Internal vulnerabilities that reduce capacity or make you more susceptible to stress	Chronic illness, perfectionism, lack of sleep, low self-compassion, unresolved trauma
Opportunities	External factors or circumstances that could help strengthen your capacity or provide support	Access to counseling, mentorship, professional growth, new routines, social connection
Threats	External stressors that can overwhelm or erode your capacity if left unchecked	Financial strain, toxic environments, high workload, major life transitions, isolation

Step 3: Reflect and Plan

- Which of your **Strengths** can you lean on more intentionally?
- Which **Weaknesses** could be supported, improved, or compensated for?
- What **Opportunities** are available right now that you could pursue to expand your resilience?
- Which **Threats** require boundaries, preparation, or protective action?

Reflection Notes:

____

____

____

____

Step 4: Identify Focus Areas

Highlight two areas from your SWOT that feel most important to address over the next few months—one you want to strengthen and one you want to protect against. Write one simple action for each:

Focus Area	Action Step	Timeline
Strength or Opportunity:		
Weakness or Threat:		

Remember: Your bucket size is not a reflection of effort or worth—it's a function of systems, biology, and experience.

By understanding it clearly, you can work *with* it rather than against it, reinforcing your strengths and building capacity where it matters most.

Input Mapping Worksheet

Purpose: To help you visualize the major stress inputs (faucets) that fill your mental health bucket. This worksheet guides you to clarify their impact, frequency, and controllability, so you can take intentional steps toward balance.

Step 1: Identify Your Inputs

List the primary sources of stress or demand currently flowing into your life. These can include external factors (workload, family, finances, health, etc.) and internal ones (self-criticism, perfectionism, fear of failure, etc.).

#	Stress Input/ Faucet	Description	Volume (High, Medium, or Low)	Frequency (Constant, Frequent, Occasional, or Rare)	Within My Control? (Yes, No, or Partially)
1					
2					
3					
4					
5					

Step 2: Analyze the Flow

- Circle three inputs that have the greatest total impact (either because they're high volume, constant, or emotionally draining).
- Place a star (*) next to any that are within your control.
- These are your first opportunities for adjustment—your valves to turn down.

Step 3: Reflect and Reframe

- Which stressors can you realistically adjust or reduce?
- Which stressors must you accept as part of your current reality?
- How might you shift your response to those uncontrollable factors?

Use the space below to summarize insights.

Reflection Notes:

____

____

____

____

Step 4: Revisit Regularly

Your flow changes with time. Revisit this map every few months or whenever you feel your bucket nearing capacity. Notice what has improved, what has intensified, and what might now be open to change.

Remember: The goal isn't to shut every faucet off—it's to understand your system well enough to manage the flow. Awareness is the foundation of control.

Drains Habit Tracker

Purpose: To help you strengthen your mental health *drains*—the habits and practices that release pressure, restore balance, and sustain recovery. This worksheet uses the cue–action–reward framework to make healthy routines more consistent and automatic.

Step 1: Choose Your Top Three Drains

Identify three key drains that, if strengthened, would most improve your mental and emotional well-being.

#	Drain Area	Why It Matters Right Now	Target Habit (Small, Specific Action)
1			
2			
3			

Step 2: Design Your Habit System

For each of your chosen drains, fill in the habit formation elements below.

Drain	Cue (Trigger)	Action (Behavior)	Reward (Immediate Benefit)	Environment (Supports/ Setup)	Habit Coupling (Attach to Existing Routine)

Step 3: Weekly Reflection

At the end of each week, check in with yourself:

- Did you practice this habit consistently?
- What helped make it easier?
- What obstacles got in the way?
- What can you adjust for next week?

Reflection Notes:

____

____

____

____

Step 4: Reinforce and Expand

After two or three weeks, reassess. Which habits are starting to feel automatic? Celebrate these wins—each one represents a reinforced drain that keeps your system flowing smoothly. When ready, add a new small habit to strengthen another drain area.

Remember: Sustainable recovery isn't built on major overhauls—it's built through small, consistent actions that keep your bucket balanced day after day.

Review Inquiry

Hey, it's Adel Elsayed here.

I hope you've enjoyed the book, finding it both useful and fun. I have a favor to ask you.

Would you consider giving it a rating wherever you bought the book? Online book stores are more likely to promote a book when they feel good about its content, and reader reviews are a great barometer for a book's quality.

So please go to the website of wherever you bought the book, search for my name and the book title, and leave a review. If able, perhaps consider adding a picture of you holding the book. That increases the likelihood your review will be accepted!

Many thanks in advance,

Adel Elsayed

Will You Share the Love?

Get this book for a friend, associate, or family member!

If you have found this book valuable and know others who would find it useful, consider buying them a copy as a gift. Special bulk discounts are available if you would like your whole team or organization to benefit from reading this. Email contact@thebucketmodel.com or visit thebucketmodel.com.

Would You Like Adel Elsayed to Speak to Your Organization?

Book Adel Now!

Adel Elsayed accepts a limited number of speaking/coaching/training engagements each year. To learn how you can bring his message to your organization, email contact@thebucketmodel.com or visit thebucketmodel.com.

References

Introduction: Time for a Rescue

1 Schaffner, A. K. (2016). *Exhaustion: A history*. Columbia University Press.
2 American Red Cross. (2017). *Lifeguarding manual.*
3 National Academies of Sciences, Engineering, and Medicine. (2019). *Taking action against clinician burnout: A systems approach to professional well-being*. The National Academies Press.
4 Panagioti, M., Panagopoulou, E., Bower, P., Lewith, G., Kontopantelis, E., Chew-Graham, C., Dawson, S., Van Marwijk, H., Geraghty, K., & Esmail, A. (2017). Controlled interventions to reduce burnout in physicians: A systematic review and meta-analysis. *JAMA Internal Medicine, 177*(2), 195–205. https://pubmed.ncbi.nlm.nih.gov/27918798/
5 Maslach, C., Schaufeli, W. B., & Leiter, M. P. (2001). Job burnout. *Annual Review of Psychology*, (52), 397–422. https://pubmed.ncbi.nlm.nih.gov/11148311/
6 World Health Organization. *Mental health at work.* (2024). [Fact sheet]. www.who.int/news-room/fact-sheets/detail/mental-health-at-work
7 Witters, D., & Agrawal, S. (2024, June). *The economic cost of poor employee mental health.* Gallup Workplace Insights. www.gallup.com/workplace/404174/economic-cost-poor-employee-mental-health.aspx
8 Shanafelt, T. D., West, C. P., Dyrbye, L. N., Trockel, M., Tutty, M., Wang, H., Carlasare, L. E., & Sinsky, C. (2023). Changes in burnout and satisfaction with work-life integration in physicians during the first 2 years of the COVID-19 pandemic. *JAMA Health Forum*, *6*(3), Article e230255. https://pubmed.ncbi.nlm.nih.gov/36229269/
9 Centers for Disease Control and Prevention. (2023). *Vital signs: Health workers face a mental health crisis, 2022.* www.cdc.gov/vitalsigns/health-worker-mental-health/index.html

10 Maslach, C., & Jackson, S. E. (1981). The measurement of experienced burnout. *Journal of Occupational Behavior, 2(*2), 99–113.
11 Demerouti, E., Bakker, A. B., Nachreiner, F., & Schaufeli, W. B. (2001). The job demands–Resources model of burnout. *Journal of Applied Psychology, (86)*3, 499–512. https://www.wilmarschaufeli.nl/publications/Schaufeli/160.pdf
12 Ursin, H., & Eriksen, H. R. (2004). The cognitive activation theory of stress. *Psychoneuroendocrinology, 29(*5), 567–592. https://psycnet.apa.org/record/2004-13940-001
13 Schaufeli, W. B., Desart, S., & De Witte, H. (2020). Burnout assessment tool (BAT): Development, validity, and reliability. *International Journal of Environmental Research and Public Health, 17(*24), Article 9495. https://pubmed.ncbi.nlm.nih.gov/33352940/
14 Liggins, O. (2021, January 21). The stress bucket—Managing your stress. Lincoln University Student Life. studentlife.lincoln.ac.uk/2021/01/21/the-stress-bucket-managing-your-stress/
15 Lowe, S. (2023, December 3). *The overflowing bucket*. It's All in the Dose. itsallinthedose.org/the-overflowing-bucket/
16 McEwen, B. S., & Stellar, E. (1993). Stress and the individual: Mechanisms leading to disease. *Archives of Internal Medicine, 153*(18), 2093–2101. https://pubmed.ncbi.nlm.nih.gov/8379800/
17 Sapolsky, R. M. (2004). *Why zebras don't get ulcers: The acclaimed guide to stress, stress-related diseases, and coping* (3rd ed.). Henry Holt.
18 Connor, K. M., & Davidson, J. R. T. (2003). Development of a new resilience scale: The Connor-Davidson Resilience Scale (CD-RISC). *Depression and Anxiety, 18*(2), 76–82. https://onlinelibrary.wiley.com/doi/pdf/10.1002/da.10113?msockid=10a8b98b81a868ca028dab1980166938

The Dimensions of a Human:

1 Guyton, A. C., & Hall, J. E. (2020). *Guyton and Hall textbook of medical physiology* (14th ed.) Elsevier.
2 Siegel, D. J. (2020). *The developing mind: How relationships and the brain interact to shape who we are* (3rd ed.). Guilford Press.
3 Goleman, D. (1995). *Emotional intelligence: Why it can matter more than IQ*. Bantam Books.
4 Dweck, C. S. (2006). *Mindset: The new psychology of success*. Random House.
5 Dweck, C. S. (2015, January 1). The secret to raising smart kids. *Scientific American*, *23*(5). https://www.scientificamerican.com/article/the-secret-to-raising-smart-kids1/

The Mass Balance Equation:

1 Libretti, S., & Puckett, Y. (2023, May 1). *Physiology, homeostasis*. StatPearls Publishing. https://www.ncbi.nlm.nih.gov/books/NBK559138/

2 42-101 Intro to BME (Spring 2005). (2005). *Topic 2: Mass balancing and kinetics in living systems*. Carnegie Mellon University. https://www.andrew.cmu.edu/course/_42-101.jalang/CourseNotes/Intro%20BME%20S05%20notes%20topic%202.pdf

Mental Health Features: The "Bucket" Model

1 Maslach, C., & Jackson, S. E. (1981, April). The measurement of experienced burnout. *Journal of Organizational Behavior*, *2*(2), 99–113. https://onlinelibrary.wiley.com/doi/10.1002/job.4030020205?msockid=10a8b98b81a868ca028dab1980166938

2 McEwen, B. S., & Stellar, E. (1993). Stress and the individual: Mechanisms leading to disease. *Archives of Internal Medicine*, *153*(18), 2093–2101. https://pubmed.ncbi.nlm.nih.gov/8379800/

3 Sapolsky, R. M. (2004). *Why zebras don't get ulcers: The acclaimed guide to stress, stress-related diseases, and coping* (3rd ed.). Henry Holt.

4 Connor, K. M., & Davidson, J. R. T. (2003). Development of a new resilience scale: The Connor-Davidson Resilience Scale (CD-RISC). *Depression and Anxiety, 18*, 76–82. https://onlinelibrary.wiley.com/doi/pdf/10.1002/da.10113?msockid=10a8b98b81a868ca028dab1980166938

The Bucket Size:

1 Engel, G. L. (1977, April 8). The need for a new medical model: A challenge for biomedicine. *Science*, *196*(4286), 129–136. https://www.science.org/doi/10.1126/science.847460

2 Borrell-Carrió, F., Suchman, A. L., & Epstein, R. M. (2004). The biopsychosocial model 25 years later: Principles, practice, and scientific inquiry. *Annals of Family Medicine*, *2*(6), 576–582. https://pubmed.ncbi.nlm.nih.gov/15576544/

3 Terenina, E. E., Cavigelli S., Mormede, P., Zhao, W., Parks, C., Lu, L., Jones, B. C., & Mulligan, M. K. (2019, May 20). Genetic factors mediate the impact of chronic stress and subsequent response to novel acute stress. *Frontiers in Neuroscience, 13*. doi:10.3389/fnins.2019.00438

4 Seah, C., Signer, R., Deans, M., Bader, H., Rusielewicz, T., Hicks, E. M., Young, H., Cote, A., Townsley, K., Xu, C., Hunter, C. J., McCarthy, B., Goldberg, J., Dobariya, S., Holtzherimer, P. E.,

Young, K. A., Noggle, S. A., Krystal, J. H., Paull, D., . . . Huckins, L. M. (2023, December). Common genetic variation impacts stress response in the brain. *bioRxiv, 27*. https://www.ncbi.nlm.nih.gov/pmc/articles/PMC10793429/

5 Likhar, A., Baghel, P., & Patil, M. (2022, August 22). Early childhood development and social determinants. *Cureus*, *14*(9). https://www.ncbi.nlm.nih.gov/pmc/articles/PMC9596089/

6 Healthy People 2030. *Early childhood development and education.* Office of Disease Prevention and Health Promotion, U.S. Department of Health and Human Services. https://odphp.health.gov/healthypeople/priority-areas/social-determinants-health/literature-summaries/early-childhood-development-and-education

7 World Health Organization. (2007, March 14). *Early child development: A powerful equalizer*. Commission on the Social Determinants of Health. https://www.who.int/publications/i/item/early-child-development-a-powerful-equalizer-final-report-for-the-world-health-organization-s-commission-on-the-social-determinants-of-health

8 Walsh, B. (2015, March 23). *The science of resilience: Why some children can thrive despite adversity.* Usable Knowledge. Harvard Graduate School of Education. www.gse.harvard.edu/ideas/usable-knowledge/15/03/science-resilience

9 American Psychological Association. (2020). *Building your resilience*. www.apa.org/topics/resilience/building-your-resilience

10 Bonanno, G. A. (2004, January). Loss, trauma, and human resilience: Have we underestimated the human capacity to thrive after extremely aversive events? *American Psychologist*, *59*(1), 20–28. https://www.tc.columbia.edu/faculty/gab38/faculty-profile/files/americanPsychologist.pdf

11 Turner, J. E., Goodin, J. B., & Lokey, C. (2024, April 20). Life's unexpected twists: Exploring the roles of emotions, motivations, self-efficacy, and secondary control following critical unexpected life events. *Journal of Research in Personality*. https://www.nu.edu/blog/lifes-unexpected-twists/

12 Mayo Clinic. (2023, December 23). *Resilience: Build skills to endure hardship*. www.mayoclinic.org/tests-procedures/resilience-training/in-depth/resilience/art-20046311

13 Marazziti, D., Fantasia, S., Palermo, S., Arone, A., Massa, L., Gambini, M., & Carmassi, C. (2024, April). Main biological models of resilience. *Clinical Neuropsychiatry, 21*(2), 155-134. www.ncbi.nlm.nih.gov/pmc/articles/PMC11129343/

14 Southwick, S. M., Litz, B. T., Charney, D., & Friedman, M. J. (Eds.). (2011). *Resilience and mental health: Challenges across the lifespan*. Cambridge University Press.

Genetic Vulnerability:

15 Collins, F. S., & McKusick, V. A. (2001, February 7). Implications of the human genome project for medical science. *Journal of the American Medical Association*, *285*(5), 540–544. https://pubmed.ncbi.nlm.nih.gov/11176855/

16 Bourque, V.-R., Poulain, C., Proulx, C., Moreau, C. A., Joober, R., Forgeot d'Arc, B., Huguet G., & Jacquemont, S. (2024, March 30). Genetic and phenotypic similarity across major psychiatric disorders: A systematic review and quantitative assessment. *Translational Psychiatry*, *14*(171). www.nature.com/articles/s41398-024-02866-3

17 American Academy of Pediatrics. (2025, December 23). *Inheriting mental disorders*. HealthyChildren.org. www.healthychildren.org/English/health-issues/conditions/emotional-problems/Pages/Inheriting-Mental-Disorders.aspx

Temperament:

18 American Psychological Association. (2018, April 19). Temperament trait. In *APA Dictionary of Psychology*. dictionary.apa.org/temperament-trait

19 ScienceDirect. Temperament. *ScienceDirect* topics. https://www.sciencedirect.com/topics/agricultural-and-biological-sciences/temperament

20 Lally, M., & Valentine-French, S. *Temperament and personality in adulthood.* Lifespan Development. https://courses.lumenlearning.com/suny-lifespandevelopment/chapter/temperament-and-personality-in-adulthood/

Chronic Medical Conditions:

21 National Institute of Mental Health. (2024). *Understanding the link between chronic disease and depression.* www.nimh.nih.gov/health/publications/chronic-illness-mental-health

22 American Psychiatric Association. (2020, November 13). *Chronic pain and mental health often interconnected.* Psychiatry.org. www.psychiatry.org/news-room/apa-blogs/chronic-pain-and-mental-health-interconnected

23 Vadivelu, N., Kai, A. M., Kodumudi, G., Babayan, K., Fontes, M., & Burg, M. M. (2017). Pain and psychology—A reciprocal relationship. *Ochsner Journal, 17*(2), 173–180. https://www.ncbi.nlm.nih.gov/pmc/articles/PMC5472077/

24 Koffel, E., Krebs, E. E., Arbisi, P. A., Erbes, C. R., & Polusny, M. A. (2016, January 16). The unhappy triad: Pain, sleep complaints, and

internalizing symptoms. *Clinical Psychological Science: A Journal of the Association for Psychological Science*, *4*(1), 96–106. https://pmc.ncbi.nlm.nih.gov/articles/PMC4928372/

25 Lim, J.-A., Choi, S.-H., Lee, W. J., Jang, J. H., Moon, J. Y., Kim, Y. C., & Kang, D.-H. (2018, June). Cognitive-behavioral therapy for patients with chronic pain: Implications of gender differences in empathy. *Medicine*, *97*(23), Article e10867. pmc.ncbi.nlm.nih.gov/articles/PMC5999451/

Socioeconomic Status:

26 Allen, J., Balfour, R., Bell, R., & Marmot, M. (2014, August). Social determinants of mental health. *International Review of Psychiatry*, *26*(4), 392–407. https://pubmed.ncbi.nlm.nih.gov/25137105/

27 Maslow, A. H. (1943). A theory of human motivation. *Psychological Review, 50*(4), 370–396. https://doi.org/10.1037/h0054346

28 Yang, Y., Niu, L., Amin, S., & Yasin, I. (2024, December). Unemployment and mental health: A global study of unemployment's influence on diverse mental disorders. *Frontiers in Public Health, 12*. https://pmc.ncbi.nlm.nih.gov/articles/PMC11672120/

Family Dynamic:

29 Coussons-Read M. E. (2013, May 3). Effects of prenatal stress on pregnancy and human development: Mechanisms and pathways. *Obstetric Medicine, 6*(2), 52–57. https://www.ncbi.nlm.nih.gov/pmc/articles/PMC5052760/

30 Ross, E. J., Graham, D. L., Money, K. M., & Stanwood, G. D. (2014, July 30). Developmental consequences of fetal exposure to drugs: What we know and what we still must learn. *Neuropsychopharmacology, 40*(1), 61–87. pmc.ncbi.nlm.nih.gov/articles/PMC4262892/

31 American Psychological Association. (2023, November 16). *High levels of maternal stress during pregnancy linked to children's behavior problems.* https://www.apa.org/news/press/releases/2023/11/maternal-stress-behavior-problems

32 McLeod, S. (2025, May 20). Attachment theory in psychology. *Simply Psychology*. www.simplypsychology.org/attachment.html

33 Erikson, E. H. (1993). *Childhood and society* (2nd ed.). Norton.

Trauma:

34 Substance Abuse and Mental Health Services Administration. (2014). *TIP 57: Trauma-informed care in behavioral health*

services. https://library.samhsa.gov/sites/default/files/sma15-4420.pdf

35 Schnyder, U., Bryant, R. A., Ehlers, A., Foa, E. B., Hasan, A., Mwiti, G., Kristensen, C. H., Neuner, F., Oe, M., & Yule, W. (2016, July 28). Culture-sensitive psychotraumatology. *European Journal of Psychotraumatology, 7*(1). https://doi.org/10.3402/ejpt.v7.31179

36 Mayo Clinic. (2024, August 16). *Post-traumatic stress disorder (PTSD)*. mayoclinic.org/diseases-conditions/post-traumatic-stress-disorder/symptoms-causes/syc-20355967

37 American Psychological Association. (2024). *Trauma*. www.apa.org/topics/trauma

38 National Institute of Mental Health. (2024). *Traumatic events and post-traumatic stress disorder (PTSD).* www.nimh.nih.gov/health/topics/post-traumatic-stress-disorder-ptsd

39 Center for Substance Abuse Treatment (US). (2014). Understanding the impact of trauma. In *Trauma-Informed Care in Behavioral Health Services, Treatment Improvement Protocol (TIP) Series, No. 57.* Substance Abuse and Mental Health Services Administration (US). https://www.ncbi.nlm.nih.gov/books/NBK207191/

Biological Deficiencies:

40 Penckofer, S., Kouba, J., Byrn, M., & Estwing Ferrans, C. (2010, May 7). Vitamin D and depression: Where is all the sunshine? *Issues in Mental Health Nursing, 31*(6), 385–393. https://doi.org/10.3109/01612840903437657

41 Coppen, A., & Bolander-Gouaille, C. (2005, January). Treatment of depression: Time to consider folic acid and vitamin B12. *Journal of Psychopharmacology, 19*(1), 59-65. doi:10.1177/0269881105048899

42 Piekiełko-Witkowska, A., Duda, M. K., Bogusławska, J., & Mackiewicz, U. (2025). The impact of autoimmune thyroid disease on cognitive and psychiatric disorders: Focus on clinical, pre-clinical and molecular studies. *European Thyroid Journal, 14*(3), Article e240406. https://doi.org/10.1530/ETJ-24-0406

The SWOT Exercise: Understanding Your Strengths and Weaknesses

43 Teoli, D., Sanvictores, T., & An, J. (2025, January). *SWOT analysis*. StatPearls Publishing. pubmed.ncbi.nlm.nih.gov/30725987/

44 Sharath Kumar, C. R, & Praveena, K. B. (2023, September 11). SWOT analysis. *International Journal of Advanced Research,*

11(09), 744-748. https://www.journalijar.com/article/46395/swot-analysis/

45 Pickton, D.W., & Wright, S. (1998). What's swot in strategic analysis? *Strategic Change, 7*(2), 101-109. https://doi.org/10.1002/(SICI)1099-1697(199803/04)7:2<101::AID-JSC332>3.0.CO;2-6

The Inputs:

The Nervous System: Your Body's Response to Stressful Inputs

1 Waxenbaum, J. A., Reddy, V.; & Das, J. M. (2025, December 1). *Anatomy, autonomic nervous system.* StatPearls Publishing. www.ncbi.nlm.nih.gov/books/NBK539845/

2 Alshak, M. N., & Das, J. M. (2023, May 8). *Neuroanatomy, sympathetic nervous system*. StatPearls Publishing. www.ncbi.nlm.nih.gov/books/NBK542195/

3 Nall, R. (2020, April 23). *Your parasympathetic nervous system explained.* Healthline. www.healthline.com/health/parasympathetic-nervous-system

Job Misalignment: When Work Becomes a Faucet with Multiple Settings

4 Maslach, C., & Leiter, M. P. (2022). *The burnout challenge: Managing people's relationships with their jobs*. Harvard University Press.

News: A High-Frequency, Often High-Volume Faucet

5 Barlow, R. (2025, October 17). *Is a news and social media overload negatively affecting your mental health?* The Brink, Boston University. www.bu.edu/articles/2025/news-and-social-media-negatively-affect-your-mental-health/

6 Li, K., Li, J., & Li, Y. (2024, April 16). The effects of social media usage on vicarious traumatization and the mediation role of recommendation systems usage and peer communication in China after the aircraft flight accident. *European Journal of Psychotraumatology, 15*(1). pmc.ncbi.nlm.nih.gov/articles/PMC11022913/

7 Lamba, N., Khokhlova, O., Bhatia, A., & McHugh, C. (2023, September 22). Mental health hygiene during a health crisis: Exploring factors associated with media-induced secondary trauma in relation to the COVID-19 pandemic. *Health Psychology Open, 10*(2),. pmc.ncbi.nlm.nih.gov/articles/PMC10517610/

8 Kellerman, J. K., Hamilton, J. L., Selby, E. A., & Kleiman, E. M. (2022, May 25). The mental health impact of daily news exposure during the COVID-19 pandemic: Ecological momentary assessment study. *JMIR Mental Health, 9*(5), Article e36966. https://pubmed.ncbi.nlm.nih.gov/35377320/

9 Mayo Clinic Press. (2024, November 12). *How the news rewires your brain.* Mayo Clinic News Network. mcpress.mayoclinic.org/mental-health/how-the-news-rewires-your-brain/

10 Huff, C. (2022, November 1). *Media overload is hurting our mental health. Here are ways to manage headline stress.* Monitor on Psychology, American Psychological Association. https://www.apa.org/monitor/2022/11/strain-media-overload

Social Media: The Double-Edged Faucet

11 Balaisis, N. (2022, December 29). The whiplash effect of social media. *Psychology Today*. www.psychologytoday.com/us/blog/our-devices-our-selves/202212/the-whiplash-effect-of-social-media

12 Naslund, J. A., Bondre, A., Torous, J., & Aschbrenner, K. A. (2020, April 20). Social media and mental health: Benefits, risks, and opportunities for research and practice. *Journal of Technology in Behavioral Science, 5*(3), 245–257. https://pmc.ncbi.nlm.nih.gov/articles/PMC7785056/

13 Palmer, C. (2023, November 1). *In brief: Limiting social media boosts mental health, the negatives of body positivity, and more research.* Monitor on Psychology, American Psychological Association. www.apa.org/monitor/2023/11/benefits-limiting-social-media

Inputs: Takeaways and Management Strategies

14 Kettering, C. *A problem well stated is a problem half-solved.* BrainyQuote. www.brainyquote.com/quotes/charles_kettering_181210

The Drains:

1 CDC, Emotional Well-Being. (2024). *Improve your emotional well-being*. Centers for Disease Control and Prevention. https://www.cdc.gov/emotional-well-being/improve-your-emotional-well-being/index.html

2 Wickham, S.-R., Amarasekara, N. A., Bartonicek, A., & Conner, T. S. (2020, December). The big three health behaviors and mental health and well-being among young adults: A

cross-sectional investigation of sleep, exercise, and diet. *Frontiers in Psychology, 11*. https://www.frontiersin.org/articles/10.3389/fpsyg.2020.579205/full

3 Bromley, K., Sacks, D., Boyes, A., Driver, C., Hermens, D. F. (2024, September). Health enhancing behaviors in early adolescence: An investigation of nutrition, sleep, physical activity, mindfulness, and social connectedness and their association with psychological distress and wellbeing. *Frontiers in Psychiatry, 15*. https://www.frontiersin.org/journals/psychiatry/articles/10.3389/fpsyt.2024.1413268/full

4 Zhang, D., Lee, E. K. P., Mak, E. C. W., Ho, C. Y., & Wong, S. Y. S. (2021, April). Mindfulness-based interventions: An overall review. *British Medical Bulletin, 138*(1), 41–57. https://pmc.ncbi.nlm.nih.gov/articles/PMC8083197/

The Nervous System: Activating Your Body's Natural Drainage System

5 Christensen, J. S., Wild, H., Kenzie, E. S., Wakeland, W., Budding, D., & Lillas, C. (2020, February 17). Diverse autonomic nervous system stress response patterns in childhood sensory modulation. *Frontiers in Integrative Neuroscience, 14*. https://www.frontiersin.org/articles/10.3389/fnint.2020.00006/full

6 Schmid, R.F., Thomas, J., & Rentzsch, K. (2024, November 4). Individual differences in parasympathetic nervous system reactivity in response to everyday stress are associated with momentary emotional exhaustion. *Scientific Reports 14*(26662). https://www.nature.com/articles/s41598-024-74873-9#citeas

Sleep:

7 Xie, L., Kang, H., Xu, Q., Chen, M. J., Liao, Y., Thiyagarajan, M., O'Donnell, J., Christensen, D. J., Nicholson, C., Iliff, J. J., Takano, T., Deane, R., & Nedergaard, M. (2013, October 18). Sleep drives metabolite clearance from the adult brain. *Science, 342*(6156) 373-377. https://science.sciencemag.org/content/342/6156/373

8 Singh K. K., Ghosh S., Bhola A., Verma, P., Amist, A. D., Sharma, H., Sachdeva, P., & Sinha, J. K. (2024, September 20). Sleep and immune system crosstalk: Implications for inflammatory homeostasis and disease pathogenesis. *Annals of Neurosciences, 32*(3):196-206. https://journals.sagepub.com/doi/full/10.1177/09727531241275347

9 Besedovsky, L., Lange, T., & Haack, M. (2019, March 27). The sleep-immune crosstalk in health and disease. *Physiological*

Reviews, 99(3): 1325-1380. pmc.ncbi.nlm.nih.gov/articles/PMC6689741/

10 Coimbra, C., de Matos, B., de Melo Faria, M., & Menezes, E. G. (2022, May 17). Repercussions of sleep deprivation on the immune system: An integrative literature review. *Research, Society and Development, 11*(7), Article e29795. https://rsdjournal.org/index.php/rsd/article/view/29795

11 Varadharasu, S., & Das, N. (2024, October 18). Sleep hygiene efficacy on quality of sleep and mental ability among insomniac patients. *Journal of Family Medicine and Primary Care, 13*(10), 4693–4698. https://www.ncbi.nlm.nih.gov/pmc/articles/PMC11610801/

Exercise:

12 Sharma, A., Madaan, V., & Petty, F. D. (2006). Exercise for mental health. *Primary Care Companion to the Journal of Clinical Psychiatry, 8*(2), 106. https://www.ncbi.nlm.nih.gov/pmc/articles/PMC1470658/

13 Mahindru, A., Patil, P., & Agrawal, V. (2023, January 7). Role of Physical Activity on Mental Health and Well-Being: A Review. *Cureus, 15*(1), Article e33475. https://pmc.ncbi.nlm.nih.gov/articles/PMC9902068/

14 Priyadarsini, A. (2024). The impact of exercise on mental health: A narrative review. *International Journal of Advances in Medicine, 11*(5), 550-553. https://doi.org/10.18203/2349-3933.ijam20242326

15 Budnick, C. J., Stults-Kolehmainen, M., Dadina, C., Bartholomew, J. B., Boullosa, D., Ash, G. I., Sinha, R., Blacutt, M., Haughton, A., & Lu, T. (2023, April 17). Motivation states to move, be physically active and sedentary vary like circadian rhythms and are associated with affect and arousal. *Frontiers in Sports and Active Living, 5*. www.frontiersin.org/journals/sports-and-active-living/articles/10.3389/fspor.2023.1094288/full

16 UT Southwestern Medical Center. (2021, March 23). *Exercise boosts blood flow to the brain, study finds.* www.utsouthwestern.edu/newsroom/articles/year-2021/exercise-boosts-blood-flow-to-the-brain.html

17 American Psychological Association. (2020, March 4). *Working out boosts brain health.* www.apa.org/topics/exercise-fitness/stress

18 Arida, R. M., & Teixeira-Machado, L. (2021, January 19). The contribution of physical exercise to brain resilience. *Frontiers in Behavioral Neuroscience, 14,* Article 626769. www.frontiersin.org/journals/behavioral-neuroscience/articles/10.3389/fnbeh.2020.626769/full

Diet:

19 Xiong, R. G., Li, J., Cheng, J., Zhou, D.-D., Wu, S.-X., Huang, S.-Y., Saimaiti, A., Yang, Z.-J., Gan, R.-Y., & Li, H.-B. (2023, July 23). The role of gut microbiota in anxiety, depression, and other mental disorders as well as the protective effects of dietary components. *Nutrients, 15*(14), 3258. https://pmc.ncbi.nlm.nih.gov/articles/PMC10384867/

20 Terry, N., & Margolis, K. G. (2017). Serotonergic mechanisms regulating the GI tract: Experimental evidence and therapeutic relevance. *Handbook of Experimental Pharmacology, 239*, 319-342. https://www.ncbi.nlm.nih.gov/pmc/articles/PMC5526216/

21 Lane, M. M., Gamage, E., Travica, N., Dissanayaka, T., Ashtree, D. N., Gauci, S., Lotfaliany, M., O'Neil, A., Jacka, F. N., & Marx, W. (2022, June 21). Ultra-processed food consumption and mental health: A systematic review and meta-analysis of observational studies. *Nutrients, 14*(13), 2568. https://pmc.ncbi.nlm.nih.gov/articles/PMC9268228/

22 Hwang, Y.-G., Pae, C., Lee, S.-H., Yook, K.-H., & Park, C. I. (2023, July 4). Relationship between Mediterranean diet and depression in South Korea: The Korea National Health and Nutrition examination survey. *Frontiers in Nutrition, 10*. www.frontiersin.org/journals/nutrition/articles/10.3389/fnut.2023.1219743/full

23 Physicians Committee for Responsible Medicine. (2026). *Food and mood: Eating plants to fight the blues.* https://www.pcrm.org/good-nutrition/food-and-mood

Substances: The "Clogs" That Impair Your Mental Health Drains

24 Mosel, S., Sharp, A., Fuller, K. (2025, March 17). *Mental effects of alcohol: Effects of alcohol on the brain.* American Addiction Centers. https://americanaddictioncenters.org/alcohol/risks-effects-dangers/mental

25 Ebrahim, I. O., Shapiro, C. M., Williams, A. J., & Fenwick, P. B. (2013, April). Alcohol and sleep I: Effects on normal sleep. *Alcoholism: Clinical and Experimental Research, 37*(4), 539-549, doi:10.1111/acer.12006

26 Webb, C. W., & Webb, S. M. (2014, April). Therapeutic benefits of cannabis: A patient survey. *Hawai'i Journal of Medicine & Public Health, 73*(4), 109-111. pmc.ncbi.nlm.nih.gov/articles/PMC3998228/

27 The BMJ. (2023, August 30). *Balancing risks and benefits of cannabis use: Umbrella review of meta-analyses of randomised*

controlled trials and observational studies, 382, Article e072348. www.bmj.com/content/382/bmj-2022-072348

28 Hill, K. (2022, June 14). *Cognitive effects in midlife of long-term cannabis use*. Harvard Health Publishing. https://www.health.harvard.edu/blog/cognitive-effects-of-long-term-cannabis-use-in-midlife-202206142760

29 Meier, M. H., Caspi, A., Ambler, A., & Moffitt, T. E. (2012, August 27). Persistent cannabis users show neuropsychological decline from childhood to midlife. *Proceedings of the National Academy of Sciences, 109*(40), E2657–E2664. https://www.pnas.org/content/109/40/E2657

30 National Academies of Sciences, Engineering, and Medicine. (2017, January 12). *The health effects of cannabis and cannabinoids: The current state of evidence and recommendations for research*. National Academies Press. https://www.ncbi.nlm.nih.gov/books/NBK425748/

Mindfulness: The Mental Drain That Grounds You in the Present

31 Fell, A. (2013, March 27). *Mindfulness from Meditation Associated with Lower Stress Hormone.* University of California Davis. www.ucdavis.edu/news/mindfulness-meditation-associated-lower-stress-hormone/

32 Calderone, A., Latella, D., Impellizzeri, F., de Pasquale, P., Famà, F., Quartarone, A., & Calabrò, R. S. (2024, November 15). Neurobiological changes induced by mindfulness and meditation: A systematic review. *Biomedicines, 12*(11). pmc.ncbi.nlm.nih.gov/articles/PMC11591838/

33 Holzel, B. K., Carmody, J., Vangel, M., Congleton, C., Yerramsetti, S. M., Gard, T., & Lazar, S. W. (2010, November 10). Mindfulness practice leads to increases in regional brain gray matter density. *Psychiatry Research: Neuroimaging, 191*(1), 36-43, https://www.ncbi.nlm.nih.gov/pmc/articles/PMC3004979/

34 Calderone, A., Latella, D., Impellizzeri, F., de Pasquale, P., Famà, F., Quartarone, A., & Calabrò, R. S. (2024). Neurobiological changes induced by mindfulness and meditation: A systematic review. *Biomedicines, 12*(11), 2613. https://www.mdpi.com/2227-9059/12/11/2613

35 Norris, C. J., Creem, D., Hendler, R., & Kober, H. (2018). Brief mindfulness meditation improves attention in novices: Evidence from ERPs and moderation by neuroticism. *Frontiers in Human Neuroscience, 6*(12), 315. https://pubmed.ncbi.nlm.nih.gov/30127731/

36 Mayo Clinic. (2022, October 11.) *Mindfulness exercises: See how mindfulness helps you live in the moment.* https://www.mayoclinic.org/healthy-lifestyle/consumer-health/in-depth/mindfulness-exercises/art-20046356

37 Imran, A. (2020, September 28). Combat against stress, anxiety and panic attacks 5-4-3-2-1 coping technique. *Journal of Traumatic Stress Disorders & Treatment, 9*(4). https://www.scitechnol.com/peer-review/combat-against-stress-anxiety-and-panic-attacks-54321-coping-technique-WiRy.php?article_id=12841

Building Lasting Habits:

38 Duhigg, C. (2012). *The power of habit: Why we do what we do in life and business*. Random House.

39 Lally, P., van Jaarsveld, C. H. M., Potts, H. W. W., & Wardle, J. (2010), How are habits formed: Modelling habit formation in the real world†. *European Journal of Social Psychology, 40*(6), 998-1009 https://onlinelibrary.wiley.com/doi/abs/10.1002/ejsp.674

40 Fogg, B. J. (2019). *Tiny habits: The small changes that change everything*. Harvest.

41 Susman, E. S., Chen, S., Kring, A. M., & Harvey, A. G. (2024, April). Daily micropractice can augment single-session interventions: A randomized controlled trial of self-compassionate touch and examining their associations with habit formation in US college students. *Behaviour Research and Therapy, 175*, 104498. https://pubmed.ncbi.nlm.nih.gov/38412573/

42 Ma, H., Wang, A., Pei, R., & Piao, M. (2023, September 12). Effects of habit formation interventions on physical activity habit strength: Meta-analysis and meta-agression. *International Journal of Behavioral Nutrition and Physical Activity, 20*(109). https://www.ncbi.nlm.nih.gov/pmc/articles/PMC10498635/

43 Singh, B., Murphy, A., Maher, C., & Smith, A. E. (2024). Time to form a habit: A systematic review and meta-analysis of health behaviour habit formation and its determinants. *Healthcare, 12*(23), 2488. https://www.mdpi.com/2227-9032/12/23/2488

The Social Connection: It Takes a Village

44 Cook, G. (2013, October 22.) Why we are wired to connect. *Scientific American*. www.scientificamerican.com/article/why-we-are-wired-to-connect/

45 Haseltine, W. A. (2025, March 25). New evidence that we're wired for connection. *Psychology Today*. https://www.

psychologytoday.com/us/blog/best-practices-in-health/202503/new-evidence-that-were-wired-for-connection

46 Martino, J., Pegg, J., & Pegg Frates, E. (2015, October 7). The connection prescription: Using the power of social interactions and the deep desire for connectedness to empower health and wellness. *American Journal of Lifestyle Medicine, 11*(6), 466-475. pmc.ncbi.nlm.nih.gov/articles/PMC6125010/

47 Reblin, M., & Uchino, B. N. (2008, March). Social and emotional support and its implication for health. *Current Opinion in Psychiatry, 21*(2), 201-205. pmc.ncbi.nlm.nih.gov/articles/PMC2729718/

48 Ozbay, F., Johnson, D. C., Dimoulas, E., Morgan III, C. A., Charney, D., & Southwick, S. (2007, May). Social support and resilience to stress: From neurobiology to clinical practice. *Psychiatry* (Edgmont), *4*(5), 35–40. https://pmc.ncbi.nlm.nih.gov/articles/PMC2921311/

49 Holt-Lunstad, J., Smith, T. B., & Layton, J. B. (2010, July 27). Social relationships and mortality risk: A meta-analytic review. *PLoS Medicine, 7*(7), Article e1000316. https://journals.plos.org/plosmedicine/article?id=10.1371/journal.pmed.1000316

50 Joo, J. H., Bone, L., Forte, J., Kirley, E., Lynch, T., & Aboumatar, H. (2022, September 24). The benefits and challenges of established peer support programmes for patients, informal caregivers, and healthcare providers. *Family Practice, 39*(5), 903–912. https://pubmed.ncbi.nlm.nih.gov/35104847/

51 Mayo Clinic. *Support groups: Make connections, get help.* Retrieved March 26, 2025, from https://www.mayoclinic.org/healthy-lifestyle/stress-management/in-depth/support-groups/art-20044655

About the Author

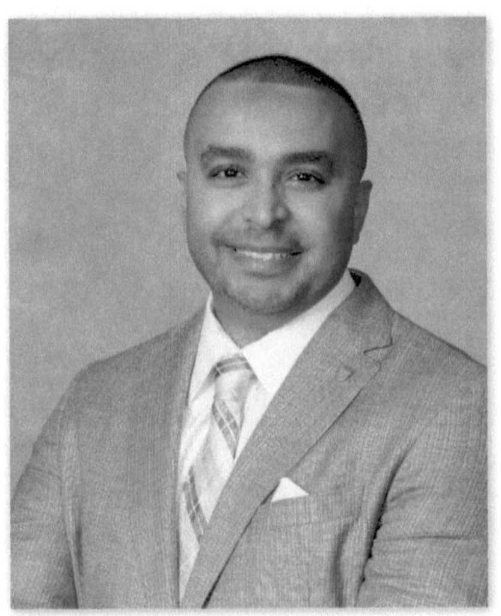

Adel Elsayed, MD, CPE, LSSBB

Adel Elsayed is a board-certified psychiatrist, certified physician executive, speaker, and assistant professor at the University of South Florida (USF) Department of Psychiatry and Behavioral Neurosciences. He provides outpatient psychiatric care and leads multiple mental health and process-improvement initiatives that support clinical excellence, operational effectiveness, and system reliability across academic and healthcare settings.

He serves as faculty for the Human Systems Engineering Scholarly Concentration at the USF Morsani College of

Medicine and contributes to interdisciplinary committees focused on safety, performance improvement, and high-reliability practices. During his clinical training, Adel received multiple outstanding teaching awards in recognition of his commitment to medical education and mentorship.

Before entering medicine, Adel worked as a process engineer and earned his Lean Six Sigma Black Belt certification from Motorola University. His statewide recognition for the top Black Belt Project in 2024 expanded his role in leading large-scale quality initiatives. He teaches quality improvement principles to medical students, residents, and fellows, integrating engineering precision with compassionate psychiatric care.

Adel can be reached at: adel.elsayed@thebucketmodel.com.

www.ingramcontent.com/pod-product-compliance
Ingram Content Group UK Ltd.
Pitfield, Milton Keynes, MK11 3LW, UK
UKHW041639190726
13854UKWH00006B/2584

9 798994 598504